Single Session One at a Time Counselling with Couples

This book introduces One at a Time (OOAT) Single Session Therapy (SST) for couples, presenting a new and innovative format for couples counselling and therapy that fills the gaps between SST and traditional couples therapy models.

The book covers the historical background of brief therapy, the concept of change in different therapy models, and the different formats of SST. The general mindset – as well as the specific thinking and practice of SST/OAAT are described in detail, combined with practical guidelines and many concrete examples from couple sessions. Five full-length OAAT session stories give the reader a clear sense of what OAAT with couples really is like and how different counsellor use their personal styles and preferences.

Single Session One at a Time Counselling with Couples is written for working therapists, therapists in training, supervisors, managers and couples themselves who are thinking of scheduling therapy.

Martin Söderquist is a licensed psychologist, licensed family therapist and couple counsellor. He has 40 years of experience of child- and adolescent psychiatry, drug abuse treatment and couple counselling, as well as training and supervision. Martin has published six books in Swedish and contributed with several articles in international journals and book chapters.

"Clients are clearly at the centre of care and work in a collaborative manner with their therapist in this approach."

Nancy McElheran, *from the Foreword*

"For many couples, individuals and families one session is what they want and need. *Single Session One at a Time: Challenge and Possibility* describes ways to help many clients in one session."

Michael Hoyt, *from the Foreword*

Single Session One at a Time Counselling with Couples

Challenge and Possibility

Martin Söderquist

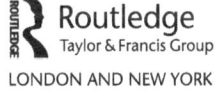
Routledge
Taylor & Francis Group

LONDON AND NEW YORK

Designed cover image: Getty Images

First published 2023
by Routledge
4 Park Square, Milton Park, Abingdon, Oxon OX14 4RN

and by Routledge
605 Third Avenue, New York, NY 10158

Routledge is an imprint of the Taylor & Francis Group, an informa business

© 2023 Martin Söderquist

Original Swedish edition published by Studentlitteratur 2020

British Library Cataloguing-in-Publication Data
A catalogue record for this book is available from the British Library

Library of Congress Cataloging-in-Publication Data
A catalog record has been requested for this book

ISBN: 978-1-032-30583-7 (hbk)
ISBN: 978-1-032-30582-0 (pbk)
ISBN: 978-1-003-30577-4 (ebk)

DOI: 10.4324/9781003305774

Typeset in Times New Roman
by Taylor & Francis Books

Dedicated To Karin my soulmate with love

Contents

Figures

Contributors

Malena Cronholm-Nouicer is a Licensed Psychotherapist, Marte Meo therapist and social worker with 25 years of experience of therapy, counselling and supervision.

Lars Dannerup is a social worker, family- and solution-focused therapist, supervisor and couple counsellor with 25 years of couple counselling in Malmö. Sweden.

Karin Wulff is a social worker and family- and solution-focused therapist with ten years of experience with drug addicts and ten years with couple counselling.

Acknowledgements

I want to thank all couples willing to share your problems and difficulties. Most of all I want to thank you for telling me your stories of managing and getting along in your lives. It has been a fantastic experience for me.

A book is a collaborative effort, and I am thankful to:

- My soul mate Karin Söderquist for her wisdom and patience
- Lars Dannerup, Karin Wulff and Malena Cronholm-Nouicer for our great collaboration characterized by respect, trust, seriousness and humour
- Bertil Ekstedt for being a pioneer companion when starting SST in Malmö and Sweden
- Bengt Weine for valuable support over the years
- Karl Tomm for inspiring generosity and curiosity to understand
- Jim Wilson for contagious energy and creativity
- Steve Harvey for sensitive and serious playfulness
- Ben Furman for being a source of inspiration over the years

I want to thank the following individuals for inviting me and my colleagues to the international network of SST, OAAT and Walk-in and for the warm and joyful welcome. I am deeply grateful for their constructive, challenging and supportive comments to my manuscript:

- Nancy McElheran for crucial encouraging and supporting in developing our work
- Michael Hoyt for giving us the chance to write two chapters in his and his colleagues' books and being a fantastic and supportive mentor with helpful comments and useful ideas
- Jeff Young for sharp proofreading and fantastic knowledge and creativity
- Flavio Cannistrà for helping us to introduce our work in Italy

Last but not least, I want to thank Simon Bloomfield for helpful and necessary linguistic reviewing.

Foreword

Nancy McElheran

This book is a first of its kind for Sweden. Martin Soderquist and his colleagues have created a "how to" book on One at a Time (OAAT) and Single Session Therapy (SST) that is a must read as it will be very useful to the therapy community across the country and elsewhere in the world.

Martin has expanded the single-session format, first implemented in North America, to his work with clients in Malmo. He offers details about the development of the OAAT/SST approach, as conceived by him and his colleagues, where couples who come to their therapy session(s) are encouraged to focus on their needs of the moment in order to get what is important from each session and then determine when and how many sessions they subsequently may want. Clients are clearly at the centre of care and work in a collaborative manner with their therapist in this approach.

Each chapter in the first section highlights a unique aspect of the One at a Time/SST approach, offering in depth understanding of the concepts surrounding the thinking that is central to its development. As Martin notes, his OAAT/SST approach is founded on concepts from the brief, single session and systemic models of therapy currently being practiced in Canada, the United States, Australia and Israel. Martin has very elegantly integrated his approach with ideas from Michael Hoyt, Arnie Slive, Monte Bobele, Moshe Talmon, Jeff Young, Karl Tomm and others in his description of the structure of a session and in creating pragmatic questions that will be useful in a session. He offers examples on how each session has a beginning, middle and end and the intervention(s) salient to each unique client situation.

Case examples are described in detail to support the learning for the reader. The ideas surrounding OAAT/SST therapy connect the reader back to the basic principles so that we can understand the evolution of this approach as well as the basic steps in conducting an OAAT couple session.

Martin and his colleagues have backed up their approach with research that corresponds with what is also known in North America: people who are in need of counselling find the OAAT/SST approach helpful, effective and empowering. No frills and low cost, OAAT/SST is proving to be a very effective way of assisting couples when they most need the help; it also eliminates wait times thereby reducing administrative costs.

Readers will find this an accessible book containing much in the way of useful, practical information.

Nancy McElheran RN MN MFT is a Clinical Nurse Specialist who provides clinical supervision and consultation at the Eastside Family Centre (EFC) of Wood's Homes in Calgary Alberta Canada. She has worked alongside colleagues at the EFC in developing the Walk-in SST approach which is now in its 28th year of operation. Walk-in SST is different from other approaches as clients walk in to the centre for a session at moments of need against making an appointment to be put on the waiting list. Nancy has authored and co-authored several articles in books and journals on the key elements of Walk-in SST.

She has had the privilege of working with Martin and his colleagues on several occasions.

Foreword

Michael Hoyt

It was with great pleasure that I accepted Martin Söderquist's invitation to write this Foreword. I first meet Martin and his Swedish team at the 2nd Capturing the Moment: Single-Session Therapies and Walk-In Services international symposium that was held in September 2015 in Banff, Canada. They presented a paper on SST with couples in Sweden, and subsequently contributed a fine chapter based on their symposium presentation to the book *Single-Session Therapy by Walk-In or Appointment*. In that paper they wrote:

> In SSCC [Single-Session Couple Counselling] you can't cover all aspects of the couple's lives. To use the session in the most effective way for the couple, the session needs to be focused on what is most important to the couple and what they can do in the nearest future. In SSCC you narrow the focus to what is most important and achievable for the couples and go deep into (or thicken) the description of goals and signs of moving in the direction of the couple's goals.

Although numerous studies had been done about single session/one-at-a-time therapy, since the original Kaiser project, until the work of Martin and his team, none had been focused specifically on the possibilities of single-session work with couples. Providing efficient help for couples – people in committed relationships – hetero- or same-sex, traditionally married or not – is a significant contribution.

One thing led to another, and it was my delight in October 2017 to visit Martin and his group in Malmö, Sweden. We had a two-day SST workshop, ate and talked together, and also played a round of golf. Alas, my play that day at the golf club was anything but "brief" or "efficient", but we, along with Swedish team member, Karin Wulff, had a fine time.

Research has repeatedly shown that a single session is the most common length of therapy. It is important to recognize that single-session therapy is not a particular theoretical approach, but rather *SST is a format or a delivery system.* "Single session" (with couples, individuals, or families) does not mean solution-focused therapy or strategic therapy or cognitive-behavioural therapy, etc., it really means approaching the session with the mind-set that *this is it*, "Let's-see-what-we-can-get-done-in-this-meeting". It's a "help today" opportunity. "One-at-a-time" does not necessarily mean there will be only one time – more sessions can be scheduled, if needed – but each session is approached as complete unto itself.

In 2019 we met again at the 3rd international SST symposium (held in Melbourne, Australia), and in 2021, Martin and his colleagues published an excellent paper called "Making the Leap with Couples in Sweden: One-at-a-Time Mindset in Action," in the book *Single Session Thinking and Practice in Global, Cultural, and Familial Contexts: Expanding Applications,* that my colleagues Jeff Young, Pam Rycroft, and I coedited. In that chapter, key portions of which are contained in the fine book you now have in hand, they described how they came to make the significant paradigm shift entailed in one-at-a-time thinking.

Especially when working one-at-a-time, therapist and client need to bring whatever is useful. To my mind, single-session therapy takes place within a "Content of Competence" where *goals* and *resources* meet via the *therapeutic alliance*. With our assistance, clients identify specific, achievable goals (giving purpose and direction to the meeting) and bring their abilities and resources to bear.

While general principles can be considered, each case is approached as unique: "one size doesn't fit all". Numerous case examples and research studies have shown that a variety of theoretical orientations have been used to produce positive one-session results. So, when things happen relatively quickly, it's an interesting challenge for researchers, what really happened, because it cannot be a gradual working-through process; something shifted more quickly.

Single-session therapy (nor any therapy) does not always resolve problems, of course, but SST works for many people. People come at the moment of their choosing, when they are ready. SST is a *minimalist constructive approach* in that it operates from the assumption that when clients feel encouraged and empowered, a small positive change often leads to larger ones – change "ripples" through the clients' internal and interpersonal systems. For many of us therapists, this has required shifting from being an Expert who "fixes" people's problems to being more of a "privileged listener" who facilitates clients' strengths and abilities to help them help themselves. One might say we move from being mechanics to gardeners.

As Martin has written, "coincidence favors the prepared mind". Approaches are more likely to be successful that emphasize patient/client abilities and positive prospects. As illustrated in the pages that follow, there are three common themes that cut across and underlie different effective SSTs: (1) mindset, (2) empowerment and (3) time. *Mindset* has to do with hope and expectation, approaching the meeting with the belief that one-session-at-a-time could be enough; *empowerment* involves the idea that clients have the wherewithal (sometimes with our facilitation) to achieve their goals; and *time* has to do with the idea that change is possible NOW.

For many couples, individuals, and families, one session is what they want and need.

Single Session One at a Time Counselling with Couples: Challenge and Possibility describes ways to help many clients in one visit. The Swedish context is both universal and specific: across the globe people want efficient help when they feel the need for assistance to resolve problems; and in every context various cultural and sociopolitical factors influence how people see themselves and their relationships, how they approach therapy, what solutions may be acceptable and available, what financial costs and other barriers may need to be overcome, etc.

The contributors to *Single Session One at a Time with Couples: Challenge and Possibility* are experts. They know the field, understand the theories and models, are human and compassionate, use the best methods and techniques, consult wisely, get good results, and write well. The procedures and many clinical cases described herein are interesting and instructive. Martin and his team have given us a wonderful gift.

Michael F. Hoyt, Ph.D. is one of the originators, with Moshe Talmon and Robert Rosenbaum, of the Single Session Therapy approach. He is the author of *Brief Therapy and Beyond: Stories, Language, Love, Hope, and Time* (2017), and has been the co-editor of three volumes about single session therapy: *Capturing the Moment: Single Session Therapy and Walk-In Services* (2014, with Moshe Talmon); *Single-Session Therapy By Walk-In or Appointment* (2018, with Monte Boble, Arnold Slive, Jeff Young and Moshe Talmon); and *Single Session Thinking and Practice in Global, Cultural, and Familial Contexts* (2021, with Jeff Young and Pam Rycroft).

Chapter 1

Introduction

Martin Söderquist

Imagine a day like any other day. You are at work as usual, and in a few moments you will meet a new couple for the first time, typical for your clinic/office.

Take a brief moment to consider each question:

- What are you thinking before session and how do you prepare?
- How do you say hello, make contact and how do you explain the context for the session?
- What is your favorite way of starting the session and establish contact?
- When the session continues – how do you think it's going and what are you focusing?
- Before ending the session – what is important to consider and do in the session?
- What are your thoughts and feelings at the end of the session?
- How do you terminate the session and how do you schedule next session?

Put this picture of your session aside before you continue with following:

Imagine the same couple coming to your first session, but they start the session by announcing they will attend only one session because the family is moving with short notice and unavailable for further sessions.

Take a brief moment to reflect over these questions:

- What are your thoughts when put in this situation?
- How do you handle the information you get and how do you subsequently start the session?
- How do you make contact and establish the possibility of a collaboration?
- What are your focus considering the different choices existing in the session?
- How do you handle all information you get when having just one to one and a half hour available?
- What are your thoughts and feelings at the end of the session?
- How do you terminate the session?

DOI: 10.4324/9781003305774-1

When you compare the two imagined sessions – what is the difference to you and to the client/couple/family and what do you think you are doing differently?

I have borrowed this Guided Imagery from Pam Rycroft and Jeff Young (Rycroft and Young, 2014). It briefly illustrates the philosophy and principles of Single Session Therapy (SST) (Talmon, 1990; Talmon, 1993) which lay the groundwork for the different session formats we now known as SST, Single Session Work (SSW), Single Session Walk-in and One at a Time (OAAT).

Let us take some moments to consider how the two different imagined sessions could have continued. Maybe the first clients[1] don´t show up to next session in spite of having scheduled continued sessions. The second clients maybe phoned a week after the session to tell that to their disappointment the move at short notice was cancelled, and now they wanted to schedule sessions. Could this have been predicted? Maybe but not very likely.

Many trials have been made over the years to assess and match clients with treatment model and predict which clients will succeed and which will not. Many trials have also been made to predict which clients will attend one session and which will attend several. These trials have not so far been very successful.

The everyday reality of clients (children, unemployment, job career, economy), unpredicted events like one partner wanting divorce, health problems and covid pandemic and much more put a lot of pressure on relationships. In recent years we have seen a growing interest in media and online for couple relationships and an increase in the number of couple scheduling counselling.

Therapists and counsellors[2] reality are also very unpredictable. The region´s or community´s economic wealth, budget cuts, political decisions and limited funds and resources create a situation where many clients are offered one assessment session and forced to wait for weeks for continued sessions and treatment. In many countries counselling and therapy is quite expensive which also contributes to couples in need of counselling being denied the possibilities.

One at a time mindset is a new way of thinking and practice; seeing every session as a new session and having the intention of doing the best of the session. The therapist is to assume the session will be the only session. When and if the client returns for another session this will be a new session with new prerequisites, new problems and new possibilities. This makes every session new, challenging and unpredictable for all involved. This perspective of the one-as-only session can be the crucial and the good start of the clients own continued work.

This is also in line with research and follow ups being done over the years saying clients expect brief contacts with counsellors, clients wanting to solve problems (Hubble et al., 1999), 30 % attend one session (Talmon, 1990) and the most common number of clients attending sessions is one, followed by two and so on (Young, 2012).

When I started working with SST I noticed a huge difference in my sessions despite the fact I had been working for many years with the idea that every session could be the last.

When assuming the session will be the only one my concentration and my focus in the session is different and my presence is closer to 100%. Here I am not thinking in terms of planning next session and continued sessions with the client. To me, the focus on being present and of being free of the thought of continued sessions as a mindset are the important gains and advantages and I think this is beneficial to the couples I see.

This book is focused on the mindset – thinking and practice – of one at a time with couples (OAAT). Couple therapy is a challenge and involves very hard work for the therapists and the couples. In combination with the thinking and practice of OAAT the challenges are even bigger but the possibilities for successful collaboration and positive outcome for the couples are great. My intention is to describe how OAAT can be achieved, organised and with particular focus on couple counselling. In the book there are many detailed examples from the session room to illustrate challenges, problems and possibilities in different contexts[3]. Most examples and quotes are from mine and my colleagues' counselling sessions with couples but I have over the years seen so many individual clients and families - they are also present in the book.

This book was originally published (2020) in Swedish (Söderquist. *Ett samtal i taget. Familjerådgivning i ny form*) and is now here restructured, rewritten and translated into English. Principles and practices presented in the book are applicable in wider social and cultural contexts, and I hope you will find the OAAT with couples thinking and the presented ideas inspiring.

Notes

1 The terms *client, couple* and *family* are used alternately depending on the context but also because the ideas in the text can be used regardless who attend the sessions. When I use the concept *couple* I mean all constellations and relationships: couple can mean the relation man-woman, same sex relations, step parents/several adults and sometimes in our couple counselling parent/parents and adult child/children.

   I also use I and we in the text. When using we my colleagues Malena Cronholm-Nouicer, Lars Dannerup and Karin Wulff are included.
2 The concepts *therapist* and *counsellor* are used alternately in the text depending on the context – therapeutic or counselling session being described. The main focus in the book is couple counselling.
3 In the first part of the book quotes and brief descriptions of sessions are from my own sessions with clients, couples and families. In later parts of the book brief and full-length descriptions of couple sessions are described by me and my counsellor colleagues.

Chapter 2

Laws and Couple Therapy Practice in Different Countries

Martin Söderquist

Psychotherapy is not a new invention. Wise people giving advice and helping others in distress and trouble has always existed. Traditionally elders, shamans, priests, doctors, philosophers, and others were the helpers, and they still are. Different therapy models, the ones we know of today, are in that sense a new Western culture phenomenon. The development of individual, family and couple therapy has in some countries been going on for a long time and in other countries has just started due to socio-economic, political and cultural factors. In Sweden and Finland, for example, it was the church that began offering couple counselling, and it was not until later that therapy and counselling were offered by communities and private organisations. The laws regulating the practice of couple therapy vary considerably from country to country. In some countries there is legislation, in some voluntary regulations and in other countries almost no laws or regulations at all. In this chapter I will try to pinpoint some similarities and differences in law and couple therapy practice in various contexts. The chapter is based on discussions with international colleagues and is not in any way meant to comprehensively cover the complex topic of legislation and couple therapy practice.

To begin with, similarities. For therapists the legal issue of confidentiality is necessary. Clients need to be certain that what is discussed with the therapist stays with the therapist. This is a ground rule of psychotherapy. At the same time therapists have to carry out risk assessments, and in some cases, confidentiality has to be retracted with the involvement of the authorities. Some clients need acute crisis intervention and/or inpatient psychiatric care, and when children are in danger of physical and sexual abuse and neglect, the therapists in most countries have to report to Child Protection Services. The need for risk assessment which involves the authorities and the need for confidentiality are involved in a delicate interplay in most countries. Couple counsellors in Sweden are mandated by law to report to Child Protection Services when they have knowledge of children being in danger. Other professionals in Sweden have to report to Child Protection Services when they suspect that children are in danger.

DOI: 10.4324/9781003305774-2

There are many differences in how psychotherapy with individuals, families and couple therapy is regulated by law and how therapy and counselling is organised.

- Cultural aspects
- Mandatory laws and voluntary regulations
- Who can practice couple therapy?
- Community or private based teams
- Costs
- Accessibility

Cultural aspects. In most countries in the world, the extended family, relatives and tribal networks are the dominant social contexts for people. Problem-solving and relationship matters are taken care of in the wider social network. Psychotherapy and counselling in the Western sense with individuals and parent – child constellations are therefore not appropriate in these cultures. Populations in many of these countries are also very poor and their main concern is how to survive wars, persecutions, poverty and starvation. One-off consultations to extended families and Single Session Therapy (SST) thinking in practice in remote places in the world are viable options here. In the books edited by Hoyt et al. (2014; 2018; 2021), there are several chapters describing SST work in contexts that are very different form the consultation room in Western societies.

Mandatory laws and voluntary regulations. When looking at this aspect it varies from no national policies and regulations at all to very stringent regulations. In most countries almost anyone can seek therapy and the only legal issue is confidentiality (Canada, the USA and the UK are examples). Complying with regulations and ethical rules decided by therapy associations are voluntary and not mandated by law.

Ireland put policies in place as late as 2016 that demands therapists to comply with regulations and ethical rules. Germany and Italy have strict regulations for therapists and in Sweden local authorities s are mandated by law since 1995 to offer couple counselling to all couples in the municipality who want that kind of help. Swedish couple counsellors are not allowed to register, diagnose or file records, and Swedish couples in counselling have the right to be anonymous. Swedish therapists working in Mental Health organisations or licenced therapists working privately are obliged to document and file records like therapists in most countries.

Who can practice therapy? In many countries anyone can practice therapy but as time goes by there is an increased need for regulations and requirements of therapists' qualifications. Germany, Italy and Sweden have strict regulations allowing only qualified therapists with a degree in psychotherapy (individual, group or family) to practice. In Sweden five years of university studies after doctoral or psychologist graduation are required to work independently as a licenced therapist. In Sweden there is no specialised university training for couple counsellors – it is integrated in the Family Therapy Program.

In Canada, the USA, Australia and European countries universities, non-profit organisations and private clinics offer therapist training. The different session formats of SST will be discussed later but the organisations where the founders worked and are affiliated with represent a broad palette. The Bouverie Centre in Melbourne, Australia is an integrated practice research centre within the School of Psychology and Public Health at La Trobe University. Woods Homes Eastside Family Centre in Calgary, Canada is a non-profit organisation. Our Lady of the Lake University in San Antonio, Texas, USA is a Catholic private University and Austin Child Guidance Centre is a non-profit-organisation. The Italian Centre for Single Session Therapy in Rome, Italy is a private organisation.

Community or private based teams. Therapy and counselling can be organised in many different ways. Therapy teams in many countries are practice centres within universities, and non-profit organisations are often funded by communities as well as by other organisations and private clinics and centres.

In the Scandinavian countries with solid social welfare systems the local communities traditionally do most of the therapy and counselling. It is the same in many other European countries. There is a growing number of private clinics and therapy centres in Sweden that offer therapy and couple counselling. Some of them have contracts with the healthcare or social services in the local community and can offer a restricted number of couple counselling sessions at a reduced fee.

Regardless how the therapy teams are organised there are challenges as well as possibilities. All organisations have their regulations and practices that frames the work of the therapists but there are always possibilities to be creative and find new ways of helping clients.

Costs. It is expensive to regularly have therapy or counselling for a long time and people seldom have the financial wherewithal. Brief therapy is requested but for many couples this might also be too expensive. There are different ways the economics of the couples can be managed: Insurance companies, local authorities, health-care centres and hospitals offering therapy and counselling to reduced fees, and with charity organisations offering legal and personal counselling. The psychotherapy reimbursement system is built on the idea of individual therapy and characterised by individualisation and medicalisation. This system doesn't accept family and couple therapy, despite all the evidence for the efficacy of family and couple therapy (Lebow and Gurman, 1995; Gurman, 2008; Hoyt and Gurman, 2012/2017). In Sweden, Finland and other countries the national health insurance will not cover the costs for couple therapy. In Sweden the law from 1995 that mandates the local authority to offer couple counselling at a reduced fee takes care of this problem. Some local communities in Denmark and Sweden, for example, offer as many as five couple-sessions for free.

Accessibility. The number of therapists could be restricted, the costs prohibitive, and the waiting lists too long which makes it difficult for couples to have therapy and counselling when they want it. Much has been done over the last years in many countries to make the situation better. Reorganising therapeutic help to people, finding new ways of seeing clients, brief therapy models being used and couple therapy online – e-mail, Zoom, Skype – to mention some efforts.

There are no restrictions for Swedish couple counsellors regarding whom they see in counselling. No matter how big or severe the problems, or how easy or difficult the goals – there are no exclusion criteria except for custody cases. These cases often involve assessments and legal processes and they are referred to a special team within the local authority. Couple counselling in Sweden is community based and is usually brief. The average number of sessions are in most teams three to four sessions: 75–80 % of all couples attend one to four sessions. Only a few stay in therapy for more than nine to ten sessions (Socialstyrelsen – Swedish National Board of Health and Welfare) (2020) Statistik. www.mfof.se/familjeradgivning/statistik.html). The statistics are most likely the similar in other Western countries.

What can SST/One at a Time (OAAT) thinking and practice offer? As already mentioned, 30% of clients – the same for couples as well as individuals in counselling in Sweden attend one session. The focus in the first and often only session for all involved must be to make their best efforts to make the session useful and constructive for the couple. This is true for all therapists and counsellors and the SST/OAAT awareness of restricted time available demands the therapist to be extra focused.

The SST/OAAT mindset can contribute to organising the services in a way that shortens the waiting lists and make therapy and counselling easily accessible to clients, families and couples. In Chapter 7 different international session formats of SST are described and how therapeutic help to clients is organised to be easily accessible.

Regardless of laws, common practices and organisation, a first session can be offered to clients, families and couples for free. For community-based teams and non-profit organisations this is possible - but not for therapists in private practice especially if they are in a OAAT mindset (no income). This first session can be called information (questions and answers), advice giving or consultation. People need to know what they may enter, start, continue with or turn down. SST/OAAT thinking and practice is a perfect fit for many couples and organisations in this respect.

A brief example: One of the partners is very hesitant and doesn't know very much about therapy and is somewhat reluctant to join his/her partner in couple therapy. After many more- or-less heated discussions the reluctant partner has agreed to attend ONE session. The first thing the other partner says in the beginning of the session is: "I think the argument that convinced my partner was when I said; 'You have the right to know more about couple therapy before you say "No" and turn it down' ".

There are many options for therapists and counsellors to invite this couple to the session. SST/OAAT thinking and practice offer a lot of ideas which will be focused on in later chapters.

To summarise: The opportunities for couple therapy as well as common practices vary a lot, owing to socioeconomic, cultural and legislative factors in different countries, with access ranging from almost non-existent to easily accessible. In many or most instances, one session is all that a couple might want or need – and SST/OAAT is ideal for meeting this need.

Chapter 3

Couple Relationships

Martin Söderquist

Many relationships begin with attraction, falling in love and a bit of madness. After a while this turns into everyday life, and intimacy and a sense of belonging deepen, but some couples are faced with problems. Romantic ideas or as Justine van Lawick (Groen and van Lawick, 2009) says "romantic illusions" of "having found the right partner", "we belong to each other for ever", "we are soul mates" and " we will always keep together" are challenged, and the partners become disappointed and frustrated. Bader and Pearson (1988) talk about the mythical match.

In every phase of the Family Life Cycle (Carter, McColdrick, 1980; 1988) there are challenges and lots of mutual decisions to make that could place stress on the relationship. When the couple can handle these crises of family development and everyday life, the relationship grows stronger.

1   Two people meet and fall in love. Often differences attract and falling in love is fantastic. Feelings of belonging, togetherness and intimacy are vital to all people and having found each other everything is in place and wonderful. There are challenges too of course. Becoming a couple needs adjustments, individual habits are challenged and new mutual behaviours in everyday life are to be found. If their families approve and accept everything is OK, but if the young couple do not get acceptance they have a harder time. All couples don't start with falling in love and acceptance by the families of origin. Some couples start with being madly in love, others grow slowly together, some couples have to take the fight to be together and others are forced together by the family of origin's cultural or religious norms.

2   Relationship deepens, and the couple starts living together. After the first period of falling in love the couple decide "we are a couple" and move in together. Being close and doing things together deepens the relationship, but there are also challenges. The partners have to find their balance of individual and couple space and time. They also have to put up boundaries around them as a couple and decide how and when to see friends and relatives.

DOI: 10.4324/9781003305774-3

3   First child is often much longed for, planned or not, and is the biggest event in life for many people and even the meaning of life for many. Becoming three and being a family is a huge step for the couple and demands adaptations of many kinds. Together they are responsible for a child 24/7, the child is first priority and this means the individuals have to step back. Life exactly as before is not possible any more. Gottman (Schwartz-Gottman and Gottman, 2015) claims that the birth of the first child causes such an adjustment to the couple's lifestyle that there is a 70% reduction of relationship satisfaction in the first year. If the couple also have to handle careers, renovating their home, problems with relatives, grandparents intruding/being over involved, death and health issues, this could challenge and place stress on the relationship. The demands can be tremendous, and couples in this phase of the family life cycle make up the majority of couples scheduling counselling in Sweden.

4   Teenage family. The growing child becoming a teenager creates a new situation in the family and demands an adjustment to new parental roles. Supporting individuation and independence, negotiation skills and balancing parental authority with trust are just some of these. The couple's relationship needs to be maintained during this phase, which can be stormy, with conflicts around parenting and adolescent behaviour.

5   Children leaving home. This gives a possibility for the couple to be on their own and do things together they have not been able to focus previously when being full time parents. The *empty nest syndrome* can hit the couple hard and the child leaving home can also react strangely (Haley, 1997). Much has been written about *baby boomers* (see Wikipedia); many couples find themselves caught in the middle, being parents to their children and taking care of their own parents.

6   Couple on their own. The experience of living a long life together, coming to rest together and with less parental responsibility can be a great reward for many couples. It gives them the chance of enjoying grandchildren. The other side of the coin is facing the death of older relatives, friends and later on with their own deaths.

In all phases of the Family Life Cycle there are constant and varied challenges for the couple in terms of autonomy and intimacy needs. The couple need to negotiate how to balance these individual and mutual needs, which are different in every phase. The couple's relationship is challenged by the different contexts all the time and in a way their relationship is under constant negotiation.

In every phase of the family life cycle there are also risks of getting stuck in patterns. Depending how the individuals react and handle the severe and overwhelming problems and stress they often fight, flight or freeze (Siegel, 1999). Two "fighters" can be a disastrous combination ending up in violent conflicts and two "flighters" run the risk of never being able to talk about and solving problems and thereby losing closeness to mention some examples.

It does not take long to establish patterns in relations, for good or bad. Habits make life easier with not being forced to always think everything over in all situations but it is not uncommon for couples to get stuck in habits. This can prevent their possibilities to discuss and solve problems. These patterns can be expressed very varied. Some couples try to change each other. What was previously attractive about the partner become disturbing, irritating, challenging and unacceptable and both partners do their best to change the other as a person or at least her/his behaviour. We all know this is impossible but it does not matter. Another pattern for couples is to constantly quarrel and fight to have the right on their side or to make decisions which in the long run can lead to violence. Often one partner is more pushy, and the other more withdrawn, referred to as *push and withdraw* pattern (Johnson 2008). Still another pattern is when one or both give up and total silence pervades the relationship. The problem with all this is that "old habits die hard", as the saying goes.

When couples find themselves in situations that they cannot handle together as well as they might wish, misunderstand each other, start fighting, stop talking and are stuck in destructive patterns, their relationship deteriorates more and more. Probably the most commonly presented problem when in therapy or counselling is the *communication problem*. This can be expressed in many ways, for example: "we don´t talk any more", "we can't discuss anything anymore","I have lost my feelings for my partner", "He/she has been unfaithful", and "we can't decide (can´t even talk about it) if we are to separate or not".

Falling in love can be easy, but when you have lived together for a while and cannot get along, separating is much harder and often destructive. In the EU nearly 50% of all marriages end up in divorce and Sweden is among the countries with highest divorce rates in Europe. The number of couples living together without being married are not included in these numbers. Last year some 62,000 children in Sweden (total population of about 10 million) had parents who were separated or in the process of separation. Many parents deal with their divorce in a non-problematic way and focus on the welfare of their children, while some struggle with negative interaction and painful memories from the couple relationship. In ten years the number of cases that end up in court in Sweden has more than doubled from some 3,200 to about 6,400. For children these court fights are the worst-case scenario.

These intense conflicts between parents put a lot of stress on the children. While they manifest high levels of stress in different ways, the consequences for the children are often so severe that a potential psychological diagnosis should not be explored until the stress levels are reduced to discern whether the symptoms are still present.

From what just has been mentioned – family life cycle crisis, relational habits and patterns, separations – it is a wonder people get along. The question of how people do manage everything in their lives and remain as a couple over many years becomes interesting. An international five-country "long term marriage" study in the 1990s was led by professor Florence

Kaslow and the Swedish part of the study was led professor Kjell Hansson and psychotherapist Ann-Marie Lundblad (Kaslow, Hansson and Lundblad, 1994). Non-clinical groups of couples married or cohabiting for more than 20 years were interviewed. Dyadic Adjustment Scale, a self-rating scale covering different aspects of marital satisfaction, and Antonovsky's Sense of Coherence Scale, a self-rating scale developed to measure coping style and increase stress-resilience capacity, were used. In the Swedish study, a comparison group of long-term marriage and cohabiting couples who had gone to family counselling was added. As expected, long-term couples describe high marital satisfaction and a high sense of coherence compared with other groups. A happy long-term relationship (married or cohabiting) can be described as an intimate relationship with someone you love, like and thrive with. Being silent together in safety and satisfaction might be the optimal sign of a good and lasting relationship. Friendship, joy, similar values, mutual activities, respect, humour, trust and loyalty are some of the important factors that increases the possibility for couples to create a long-term relationship. According to Gottman (1994) there are three groups of couples that stay together 1. Volatile. Couples who sometimes quarrel and remain passionately involved with each other. 2. Validating. Compatible, supportive and appreciative. 3. Avoidant. Living parallel and somewhat separate lives. (See also Wallerstein and Blakeslee, 1996).

If falling in love often is fairly easy, and opposites attract, staying together for a long time requires a lot of investment in the relationship, hard work of adjusting to each other and together going through crises and problems.

How can therapy and counselling be of help for couples and families when going through crisis and handling problems? The different therapy models, brief therapy and the historical background of One at a Time counselling will be presented in the following chapters.

Chapter 4

Change or Not – That is the Question

Martin Söderquist

"The important shift from individual to relational mindset was introduced by family therapy pioneers like Erikson, Satir, Minuchin and Haley in the 1960–1970s (see Satir,1967; Haley,1973, 1976; *Minuchin, 1974*). This had an enormous impact on the field – clients were seen in their social context and family members were accepted as important and helpful to the clients."

(Söderquist et al., 2021)

Change is a concept recurrent in all therapeutic models and discussions of therapy, counselling and consultation. All the models existing today are aiming to help clients, couples and families think differently or do something different; bring them increased understanding and knowledge of themselves and others and giving them the chance of processing their feelings.

Some years ago I put together a summary of different therapeutic models focusing relational models – not models grounded in individual thinking. My purpose was to understand similarities as well as differences between the models. I do not claim this summary to be comprehensive and the summary is presented as the way I saw the models by that time. I added Couple Therapy models later.

Structural / Strategic family therapy – First order cybernetics

Originator	*Satir*	*Minuchin*	*Haley*
Model	Communicational Family Therapy	Structural Family Therapy	Strategic Family Therapy
Definition of problem	Incongruent, unfree communication	Organization of family system, symptom has a function (Boundaries)	Organization of family system, symptom has a function (Hierarchy)
Definition of change	5 Freedoms	Change of boundaries	Reestablish hierarchy
Role of therapist	Sculptor	Director	Paradoxical scientist

Figures 4.1–4.7 Definition of problem, change and role of therapist in 12 different therapeutic models[1]

DOI: 10.4324/9781003305774-4

Bried Therapy – Mental Research Institute

Originator	*Watzlawick, Weakland, Fisch*
Model	Mental Research Institute Brief Therapy/ Problem Solving Therapy
Definition of problem	Attempted solution to problem becomes the problem
Definition of change	First order change – change within the system Second order change – change of change
Role of therapist	Out of the box challenger

Structural /Strategic familjetherapy – modern originator

Originator	*Alexander*	*Henggeler*
Modell	FFT/ Functional Family Therapy	MST/ Multi Systemic Therapy
Definition of problem	Problem / symptom has a function in the family system	Social-ekological model. Multiple causes to problem
Definition of change	Change patterns of communication & structure, reframing	Change interaction in the families and their interaction with other systems
Role of therapist	Pilot	Man-to-man marker

Systemic family therapy – Second order cybernetics

Originator	*Palazzoli, Cechin, Boscolo*
Model	Systemic family therapy – Milano model
Definition of problem	Rigid, stuck family system. Symptom has a function in " the family game"
Definition of change f	P: Invariant prescription C & B: Circular questions
Role of therapist	P: Humble manipulator C & B: Gurus of questions

Couple therapy models

Originator	*Johnson*	*Gottman*
Model	EFT/Emotionally Focused Therapy	Gottman Evidence Based Couples & Marital Therapy
Definition of problem	Patterns of attachment	Negative patterns of interaction. The four horsemen of Apocalyps
Definition of change	Understand relational patterns – create new experiences	Help couples solve conflicts and repair/build friendship and love. House of Sound Relationship
Role of therapist	Engine-driver	Integrator of research, training and therapy

Figures 4.1–4.7 (Cont.)

Language systemic & Narrative models

Originator	Anderson & Goolishian, Tom Andersen	White
Model	Language system	Narrative
Definition of problem	Problem defining system	Problem saturated narrative
Definition of change	Open up, generate new information, create meaning	Reauthoring; deconstruct and create new narratives
Role of theraoist	Conversational expert	Partner – against problem - for creating new narratives

Solution Focused Bried Therapy – something quite different

Originator	De Shazer, Kim Berg
Model	SFBT
Definition of problem	No ideas of problems, pragmatic model
Definition of change	Create decriptions of clients goals and exceptions, build solutions
Role of therapist	Taxi driver / "Leading from behind"

Figures 4.1–4.7 (Cont.)

All models share the focus on relationships in contrast to previous individual models.

The differences are about how problem, change and the role of therapist are seen.

Many of the models are in a way quite similar – the client experiences a problem that therapy can or will solve. Depending on the theoretical orientation of the therapist different aspects of client's lives are noticed and reinforced. There are differences of course. One of them is the aspect of time – how much time will change take according to the models. Another one is if the client needs to understand and process his/her problems, which takes time, or if the client can solve problems by doing something different. A third difference is if the client and therapist need to build attachment and safety in their relationship over time or if the constructive alliance begins immediately.

The most crucial difference between models is how the therapist see the resources and abilities of the client. Is the client capable of handling things on his/her own or is the therapist the expert knowing what the problem is and how it can be solved? One at a Time (OAAT) counselling is a session format that is built on the assumption that clients are competent and their own expert. Clients can choose what is best for them when it comes to goals of sessions and what format for sessions.

Three questions arise here:

- Are all clients/couples willing to make a change?
- Are all clients/couples willing to make the change proposed by the therapist?
- Is it really necessary to make changes?

When talking about changes in this context most people see this as a personal change. If the goal of therapeutic and counselling sessions is a personality change, we can directly and frankly say: "Many clients are not interested in changing themselves". They want to preserve their dignity and integrity and they express this in different ways: Some say their partner is the one that has to change – if he/she said or did this or that everything would turn out differently. Others say the pressure from other people or circumstances is the problem and that has to be changed. Others say they cannot think or do differently because they have always seen, thought and done things in a certain way and they are not willing to change that.

When a person, a couple or a family for some reason end up in the session room with a therapist, he/she/they might not be interested in changing as a person. For their part, the therapist might be working according to his/her preferred therapeutic model to produce change in the client. Solution Focused Brief Therapy concepts *customer, complainant and visitors* are applicable here. As a result of the session customers see their problems and are willing make to make an effort to change, complainants see the problems but want others to make the necessary changes and visitors just want to visit the session (de Shazer, 1988). Eastside Family Centre group changed complainant to surveyor, a more solution focused language (personal communication, Nancy McElheran).

In most cases they together find a way of working together that is beneficial to the client. Most therapists respectfully talk to all reluctant and "unmotivated" clients without being too pushy or forcing. Reluctant and "unmotivated" clients, as everyone else, have hopes, dreams and goals that can appear when talking in the session. In other cases, the therapist has to accept the fact that the client in that moment is not interested in the therapy/counselling the therapist suggests. There might be many reasons for the client's decision such as working alliance and collaboration did not work, or the session was not what they expected. These reasons are most often in no way related to the competence or capability of the client or the therapist.

Do the clients really have to change as persons? Is it not enough to think or do something a little bit different? Often clients and therapists end up in an agreement of this - despite their differences and the pressure from the client's network and from the therapist's model. The thinking and doing can be done at once or later. I have many times heard myself say approximately like this: "You don't have to change as a person but it is not a law of nature always to think and do in a certain way. Sometimes it is enough to think or do a little bit different as a first step on your thousand-mile journey". If the couple has given a small example of thinking/doing differently this can be focused and their descriptions can be made thicker and wider. If the couple has not given an example, my little talk can bring the session in the direction of what could be small and different for the couple.

Reflection time

Take a brief moment think through these questions:

1 From the point of view of your preferred therapeutic model – what is change and how is change accomplished?
2 How have you made changes in your own life?
3 When comparing the two pictures – what similarities and differences do you see?

This brief exercise is also borrowed from Rycroft and Young (2014) and most often show change can be accomplished in many different ways. It also brings up the question if therapeutic changes in sessions are quantitative or qualitative. From a theoretical standpoint quantitative and qualitative changes or expressed differently – first and second order changes (Watzlawick, Weakland and Fisch, 1974; Watzlawick, 1978) are different. First order change is a change within a given system and second order change is changing the system (doing things in the dream compared to going from dreaming to waking). Development is often gradual (quantitative) but crucial steps are taken suddenly (qualitative).

Some examples:

The little child struggling with trying to walk but is for the moment only capable of standing still – but suddenly he/she is capable to take a step or two. An older child fights with the letters to learn how to read – suddenly he/she begin to read a word or two. A man has for a long time been thinking of something back and forth and one morning he wakes up and the first thing is to say to himself: I am going to do it now. A woman cannot decide if she should separate from her partner or not; she has talked to her friends without coming to a decision. One day she sees her daughter playing in the backyard and begins to imagine her daughter two years older and then she knows.

When talking about therapy, music and other contexts the concept *pivot chord or pivotal moment* (Rosenbaum et al., 1990) is often used to escribe a precise point in time when something appears obvious, suddenly changed and absolutely crucial. These moments resembles the concept turning points used in drug and addiction research. Persons who are able to stop abusing often report they fell in love with someone for real, found God or something else very great and meaningful.

Afterwards both clients and therapists can remember and point out such pivotal moments in their sessions (Söderquist, 2009b, in Swedish). The following quotations describes this: "When the therapist told me that I managed more than I thought I knew directly what to do", "When we talked about ... in the session I suddenly knew what to do", "I will never forget when grandma began crying in the session – after that session I haven't used heroin".

The problem with pivotal moments is that they are very hard to plan and deliberately create. The client and therapist might both work hard to get to these pivotal moments, but it is not until afterwards the therapist can know if what was said and done in the session was useful and crucial for the client.

This excerpt from one of my couple OAAT sessions illustrates this:

When we have been talking for some time, I still do not know if the couple are telling me they are to separate or if they both want to work for enhancing their relation. I try to use clarifying questions but this does not give me a clue. It seems like the woman wants divorce but not the man. They have not discussed that and they are both unsure and do not know what their partner thinks. As a way to get away from the situation of talking in circles without getting anywhere I suggest an exercise to both: "Reach out your hands in front of you, look at them and imagine a picture of your separation in one of the hands and in the other hand you put your picture of continuing as a couple. Look carefully at both hands one at a time and go find the picture and when you have done that close your eyes. When opening your eyes again lay both hands on your breast and ask yourself: Which hand is closest to my body?"

Both turn to each other and simultaneously and laughingly they say: "separation". This was very unexpected to me, and I can just say: "Are we where you wanted to be in the session?". They both agree. We continue the session with a discussion and their plans for how to do the separation. They seem to be in agreement and relieved".

It is not only clients experiencing pivotal moments. Therapists and counsellors can also experience these moments. For me and my colleagues a visit to an out-patient clinic in the USA many years ago is a memory not easily forgotten:

During the visit to the clinic we had pictured ourselves meeting colleagues, being behind the mirror in the observation room as team members and by this learning a lot. It turned out we on several occasions were asked to do consultation interviews – interviewing clients and their therapists about their sessions. We were really in the hot spot and we were not that experienced by that time. One of our American colleagues, Mike, had met the couple for five or six sessions. The man was sentenced by the court to 75 hours of therapy for the second time, having been convicted of addiction and drug-related criminality. Mike wanted me to do a consultation interview – he saw the sessions at a standstill: "We are not getting anywhere, the guy is just sitting off time and I have to meet him and his wife 70 more hours! (Korman and Söderquist, 1994. You can find the full session in transcription in English and free download on: www.sikt.nu).

To me the session was an ordinary consultation but to Mike it turned out to be crucial. In the end of the session Mike seemed to have changed his mind. In spite of what he had told me before the session, Mike could give me and the couple many examples of how the couple impressed him and what he saw them doing.

After the session Mike told me: "When you early in the session asked the couple what I had been doing that was good for them I froze to ice and thought that they were going to say "nothing" (they definitely did not). Mike continued: The guy spoke a lot today more than he had for five or six sessions. That is fantastic. Now I think the couple has come a long way, they have done so much I do not know what to talk about in the next 70 sessions.

Another example:

Anna had a very problematic upbringing and background and suffered from psychosis and depression. She did not want to see anyone from the Psychiatric clinic and scheduled an appointment with the Outpatient team Avenboken, (a solution-focused team run by the Social department of the community) where I worked as therapist at the time. Anna met one of my colleagues and wanted for some reason see me for a session. My memory of this session is very strong and vivid. When we are about to begin the session, Anna walks around in the room looking for invisible microphones she is convinced are hidden everywhere. She seems to be stressed when a car passes by outside the window. After a while she sits down. After welcoming her, I suggest the following: You have already had a first session with my colleague, and we do not have to do that again. You know what you want, you are the expert about yourself, and you know yourself. My suggestion is you interview me to inform you what you need to know to be able to trust me. I won't ask you anything.

I will never forget what happens after this: Anna straightens up, look me in the eyes (she had not until now) and she begins making a very impressing and focused interview. It lasts for 30 minutes, and she asks me important and relevant questions, and at the same time she shares some information about her own life. On no occasion do I need to say "I don't want to talk about that". Anna's transformation from a frightened, suspicious and unbalanced person to a very capable and effective person controlling the situation was the most impressive and fantastic I had ever experienced. When we terminated our sessions after a year, we wrote a chapter in a Swedish book (Söderquist, 2003).

We had no agreement on therapy form the start, just one session, and this was a pivotal moment for both of us. Anna returned for several sessions later on, and every session was definitely a new one.

Change is a varied concept, and we all have our own definitions. Change can be made in so many ways – I usually think and say "Problem descriptions are very much alike and in the long run boring". But when people describe how and what they did to solve their problems their stories are unique and unexpected. This is what makes therapeutic sessions so interesting.

Let us now turn to couple therapy and counselling.

Note

1 Satir, 1964; Minuchin, 1974; Minuchin and Fishman, 1981; Haley, 1973; 1976; Watzlawick, 1978; Watzlawick, Weakland and Fish, 1974; Alexander and Parsons 1973; Hengeler et al., 1994; Sexton and Alexander, 2003; Selvini Palazzoli, Boscolo, Cecchin, Prata, 1978; Schwartz-Gottman & Gottman, 2015; Johnson, 2008; Andersen, 1991; Anderson, 1997; White, 1989; de Shazer, 1982, 1988,1991; de Shazer et al., 2007; Berg and Miller, 1992; Berg and Dolan, 2001; George, Iveson and Ratner, 1999; Ratner, George and Iveson, 2012.

Chapter 5

Couple Therapy and Counselling

Martin Söderquist

The pioneers of family therapy focused theories and practices on families. Couples were not the main interest from the start and marriage therapy and marital counselling were seen as "the ambivalently embraced stepchild of family therapy" (Gurman, 2010). Couple therapy is nowadays a specialist branch. Various definitions of couple therapy include psychotherapeutic interventions, techniques, strategies and methods to help intimate partners reduce stress and increase relationship satisfaction. Therapy is often used to describe deeper and broader personal work including several or long-term sessions agreement between couple and therapist. Counselling is described as problem solving, focusing on smaller goals and often fewer sessions. Sometimes therapy and counselling are used alternately.

The question of intention and effect is also interesting in this context. Sometimes ordinary/social conversations have therapeutic effects (talking to a friend or relative) and sometimes therapeutic or counselling sessions intended to help clients do not do that or even have iatrogenic effects, that is negative effects exacerbated by interventions.

There are many challenges for couple therapists and counsellors to handle. The partners often want a judge to agree and side with them against their partner. Neutrality is recommended but not always easy to uphold. Another challenge is when the couples flood the session with all their problems, and these can be of life and death character (their relationship continuing or dying). A third challenge are the social, political and economic changes over the past few decades. The consequences of these changes invite therapists and counsellors to be informed, enlightened and trained in gender, racial, migration, refugee and global issues. There are also multiple ways of being a couple – married or not, cohabiting or not, same or different sex and polyamorous relationships are some examples.

Many couple therapy models have been developed, most of them problem focused and integrative in practice. Gurman (2010) mentions six major types or traditions of couple therapy based on different theories: behavioral, humanistic-existential, integrative, psychodynamic-transgenerational, social constructionist and systemic.

DOI: 10.4324/9781003305774-5

It is not the scope of this book to go into all these models but couple therapy models can also be described by the following three points:

The therapist as expert or non-expert. Understanding problem and focusing emotions and cognitions or describing different situations and focusing doing. Sessions focusing on past-present or future.

Of course, the counselling sessions will be very different if the counsellor focuses past or present problems or preferred future, positioning her-/himself as expert, conversational host, teacher or sensei. Common factors research (Wampold and Imel, 2015) and the Dodo Bird effect (Hubble et al., 1999) has shown all therapy models more or less equally effective and giving positive results for the clients. The therapy models can be seen as important to the therapists as a map or navigator in the sessions, and we all have our personal preferences.

In my colleagues and my version of Single Session Therapy (SST)/One at a Time (OAAT) with couples our thinking and practice include a preference for therapist as non-expert, focusing doing and present-future most of the time. Sometimes couples present problems that need more attention than just being mentioned and the couples are in the front seat – we are to follow their lead. The focus in the OAAT session will still be on present situation and hopes for the session. SST/OAAT is very different from many couple therapy models which often are grounded in theories, problem focused and built on several sessions. The thinking and practice of OAAT with couples will be described in detail, including no serial thinking and focusing the session today, in later chapters of the book.

When focusing the session today and the couple's hopes the couple therapy challenges are easier to handle – not taking sides or judge and not trying to solve all problems.

Some of the therapeutic models for working with couples are more popular and influential than others internationally and in Sweden. In our team we have in our personal ways integrated OAAT with:

Gottman Method Couples Therapy: This model integrate research, training (psycho education) and therapy helping couples replace negative interactions/ patterns of conflicts with constructive patterns of interaction. The Sound Relationship House is a summary of important research being done over the years by Gottman. The House gives the couples the tools to build a happy and healthy relationship. The weight-bearing walls of trust and commitment and the six levels of the house help the couples create a solid bond. Floor one is Build Love Maps – the firm foundation of knowing each other (an essential guide to the partners inner world). Floor two is Sharing Fondness and Admiration. Floor three is Turning Towards (instead of Away or Against). Floor four is The Positive Perspective. Floor five is Manage Conflict (knowing what to do when unavoidable conflicts start or escalate). Floor six is Make Life Dreams Come True (help each other to do what it takes to make that happen). Floor seven is Create Shared Meaning (build an inner world as a couple). As when building a house, a relationship and therapy need to start with foundations, groundwork and walls and then adding floor upon floor (Schwartz-Gottman and Gottman, 2015; www.gottman.com).

Emotionally Focused Therapy (EFT): Grounded in systems theory and attachment theory Sue Johnson has developed EFT focusing adult attachment while the other originator Leslie Greenberg has developed EFT in the direction of processing of emotions. The goal of therapy is for the couples to understand their relationship and underlying emotions/feelings. By this understanding, they are able to turn to each other and create a safer relationship. In EFT sessions client and therapist work together in exploring the couple's interaction and exploring internally their feelings, emotions and thoughts. Naming and accepting underlying emotions and attachment needs/fears and facilitate each person's expressions directly to their partner (external communication) make it possible to create a safer relationship. The EFT process is divided into phases and requires 16 sessions. EFT strongly emphasises the importance of the therapeutic alliance and of the therapist as a safe base (Johnson, 2008; Grennberg, 2008).

Narrative Therapy: All humans create stories and narratives of themselves and of life in general. These narratives can turn into thin, limited, problem saturated and destructive narratives in problem situations. The goal in narrative therapy is to widen the narratives of clients, make the narratives thicker and more constructive to the clients. Couples and therapist are collaborative co-researchers and widen their research to cultural, power and political narratives by distancing and taking a position in relation to problems. Unique outcomes and moment of connection are focused by externalizing conversations and scaffolding questions. (White, 1989; Asplund Ingemark et al., 2013; Gurman, 2010).

Solution Focused Brief Therapy (SFBT): This model represents a different paradigm. Unlike other models, it contains no theory of problem and their causes and see no relation between problem and solutions. SFBT is a pragmatic model of therapy – the model is developed and developing collaboratively with the clients. The focus in sessions are descriptions of pre-session change, hopes and goals of the client and their future direction. The role of the therapist is to remind the client/couple about this. Through this different focus the "problems are dissolved" when client and therapist are building the couple's solutions. The therapists are "leading from behind" – inviting couples to describe their preferred future and following the couple's lead closely (de Shazer et al., 2007; Berg and Miller, 1992; Berg and Dolan, 2001; Korman and Söderquist, 1994).

The therapy models nowadays are more or less brief, and in the following chapter we focus on brief therapy.

Chapter 6

Brief Therapy

Martin Söderquist

> "Next shift in mindset, in the 1980–1990s, was to brief relational work. De Shazer (1985, 1988), Kim Berg (Berg and Dolan, 2001), Hoyt (1994, 1996, 1998), White (White and Epston, 1990) and many others were leading proponents."
>
> (Söderquist et al., 2021)

We are all influenced by what we have learned and/or what we are used to.

Here is an example:

Lotta came running into the *standing office* (literally no chairs; all meetings were supposed to be very brief) of the Swedish Public Employment Service. She was recently unemployed and wanted help to find a new job. Eva met Lott and their meeting was very brief – just a few minutes. In this short time they got to know each other a bit and Lotta told Eva what she wanted. Eva was in a training group to learn how to do sessions and meetings in a solution-focused way and asked Lotta if she was interested in being interviewed by a consultant (I, Martin Söderquist) and get his and the training group's comments and ideas. Lotta said yes immediately.

The interview was some days later and Lotta received a lot of encouraging comments and ideas. After the interview the group of workers and I had a discussion and many of them were quite pessimistic of Lottas chances to get a job. They said she wasn´t concentrated, all over the place and seemed to have a lot of problems. I, being a psychologist and family therapist, and the one doing the interview thought, "Have we met the same person?" I was surprised and did not get what had given rise to all this pessimism. I had talked to a thoughtful Lotta, who described what she wanted, her plans for the future, and how people who knew her would notice her progress. Paradoxically, the training group saw all the problems, and the psychologist saw her possibilities.

Next time we met in the training, Eva told us that Lotta had phoned her and thanked for the help that she got, and she had already begun a new job.

We are all influenced by what we learned when growing up, in school and later on in higher education. We see and hear what we are looking for and think what we have learned. Different therapeutic models are extremely

DOI: 10.4324/9781003305774-6

helpful as guidance and a map to orient and plan the sessions, but the models could and should not be some kind of truth. "The map is not the territory" is often referred to in the literature. Theories and models help us notice, see and hear what the clients tell us but can also mislead the therapist in a direction not wanted by the clients. Cecchin (1993) talked about not falling in love with your own model and the importance of being irreverent to your own model to be able to be sensitive and open. In the solution-focused model, the concept of "solution forced" (Nylund and Corsiglia, 1994) is when the therapist works hard to use exception and future questions, while the client has a feeling of "I cannot talk about my problem here". In all therapeutic models this duality of possibilities and risk exist.

Hoyt (2017, p.207) points out three criteria for evaluating therapeutic models:

- *Effectiveness*: Does the model work? Does it give results?
- *Aesthetic*: Is the model interesting and attractive?
- *Ethical*: Is the model respectful to the client? Does it help the client grow?

Brief therapy and Context of Competence

Single Session Therapy (SST) began from findings of statistical facts showing that 30% (Talmon, 1990) of all clients attending only one session and one session being the most common number of sessions for therapists. The session formats also have a theoretical background in *brief therapy*.

Brief therapy originated from Milton Erickson's work especially his *utilisation principle* (Haley, 1973). What the client brings to the session – resources, problems descriptions and goals – are used to help the client. Erickson used hypnosis and paradoxical interventions in ways that many therapists didn't understand but he did it very effectively. Paradoxical interventions are, according to the Swedish therapists Olson and Petitt "interventions made by the therapist simultaneously in two different and contradictory levels to produce wanted changes regardless of what level the clients answer are" (Olson and Petitt, 1999, author's translation).

A great number of books have been written about how Erikson worked for example *Uncommon therapy* by Jay Haley (1973) and *A teaching seminar with Milton H. Erikson M.D.* edited by Jeffrey Zeig (1980). Erikson's work was unique, inspirational and is the source of many models of family therapy and brief therapy and they can all be seen as brief models.

Hoyt specifies the characteristics of brief therapy (Hoyt, 2017, p. 205):

- The development of rapid and positive alliance
- A focus on specific, achievable measurable goals
- The clear definition of client and therapist responsibilities
- An emphasis on strengths and competencies

- The introduction of novelty, assisting the client toward new perceptions and behaviours
- A here-and-now (and next) focus on the present and future more than on the past

I want to add:

- Big problems do not always need big solutions
- Aim of session is to help the client help himself/herself
- Respect of the goals, competencies and limitations of the client

The focus of brief therapy on few sessions can also be pointed out. Solving problem does not necessarily take a lot of therapeutic sessions over time. Another focus is action, focusing on behaviour and handling of things and the fact that life itself is the grand master not therapy.

Follow ups and evaluations show (see Hubble, Duncan and Miller, 1999) clients expect brief contacts/sessions. They also show clients attend a few sessions and numbers from Couple Counselling in Sweden show that 75–80% attend one to four sessions, changes occur in the beginning of therapy/counselling (sometimes in the first and only session) and brief therapy is quite as effective as long-term therapy. We know that up to 70% of the positive results can be explained by the clients´ own resources and the client-therapist alliance. The therapeutic model and placebo effect explain minor parts. According to Hubble, Duncan and Miller (1999) the model and placebo effect explain only 30% of the results (15% each).

In later publications Miller and Bertolino have reported that 80–87% of the difference between client in treatment and clients with no treatment can be explained by client and non-therapeutic factors and 13–20% of a positive result can be explained by treatment. (Miller and Bertolino, 2012, pp. 22–23).

Common factors research (see Wampold, 2001; Wampold and Imel, 2015) have for many years showed the similarities of different therapeutic models – these similarities are more important than the models in explaining positive results in therapy.

In a project Lee, Uken and Sebold (2003) came to the conclusion that a client's readiness to change was not particularly crucial which was rather surprising. However, detailed and concrete goals and client and therapist in agreement on these goals was crucial (Lee, Uken and Sebold, 2007; Lee, Sebold and Uken 2003).

Flavio Cannistrá (2021) presents his own choices to be briefer in therapy. Be pragmatic, be efficient, avoid reification and adopt a multi-theoretical mindset. This requires an open mind, humility and a strong desire to learn more.

All being said so far can be summarised in what Hoyt calls *context of competence* (Hoyt, 2014; 2017; 2018): In brief therapies clients and therapists co-create a context of competence when Goal, Resources and Alliance overlap and intersect. Effective therapy involves all three.

Different contexts. As therapist and client, you are always in different contexts and the context of competence model can be applied in different contexts and situations. The contexts influence what we do and what our possibilities are. If we are working in outpatient or hospital units, in school or in social service this decide what our directives and specific roles are. There is always a context in which clients and therapists have sessions. Clients and therapists most often come from different background and have varied worldviews, and this must also be negotiated, coming to terms with and agreed on.

These contexts have to be very clear for both parts which the following brief story relates:

A colleague of mine had a session with a family referred from Child Protection for assessment but when they came to session, they thought they were going to get some help – their social worker had said that. My colleague immediately had to tell them he had been asked to make an assessment of the parents' abilities to take care of the children and guarantee their safety. The parents didn't know this in advance.

Resources and competencies. Noticing and focusing these highlights and reinforce what the client already has done and is doing. You do not have to cross the river to get to water instead you can build on what there is. The resources and competencies of the client are what most of all are responsible for positive results. (Hubble, Duncan and Miller, 1999). Telling the client: "You are more successful than you know" is maybe what the client needs to hear most of all. I have borrowed this expression from Dan Gallagher, an American therapist. It is his favourite expression (Gallagher, personal communication, 1992.) It is sometimes important and hard to notice and affirm the resources and competencies of the client to empower the client which can be seen in the following excerpt:

Cilla, 16 years old, was helped by an outpatient clinic nurse to contact child and adolescent psychiatry after having been attacked and raped. She told the nurse it was OK for her to see a male therapist and she said she could go to the clinic where I was – another part of the city (I offered to come to where she was). Cilla was low and scared, and it was obvious to everyone how bad she felt. My first question to her was: "What are you good at?". Cilla was silent for a long time and then she said: "Nothing – I didn't even finish school". I began regretting my first question but chose to continue my line of thinking by asking her: "If your mother was here today – what would she tell you are good at?". Cilla thought for a while and said: "Nothing" and added "Well, she would tell I am very good at shouting". I was getting worried that the more of these kind of questions and answers there were, the more the session would confirm Cilla's negative self-image and her experienced failure. I was thinking – there must be someone somewhere being able to say something positive about Cilla. I asked her about friends (she did not have many), boyfriend (did not want to talk about him) and teachers (she was not attending school). Now I was really getting worried for.

Finally Cilla suddenly said: "I know now. When in middle grade school (ten–12 years old) my teacher was the best teacher I ever had". I was relieved and said: "If that teacher was here today what would he/she said you are good at?". Without any hesitation Cilla said: "Cilla is competent, energetic and interested." I asked her: "What advices would the teacher give you in your situation at this moment in your life?" Cilla immediately said: "Go out and live as you usually do and talk to your mother". The first advice – going out and live normally – Cilla saw as a good one, but she was reluctant to the second piece of advice. Later in the session Cilla came up with things she had have the energy and guts to do like telling the police, standing up to her mother and stepfather and how she was asserting herself in different contexts. Before finishing the session, I summarised what I had heard her telling me in the session. Most of all I pointed out her strengths. Cilla commented and this is the best summary: "When someone believes in me – I have the energy and endure.

An example from a couple session:

The husband was very worried when his wife after their first child was born seemed to be without any energy and seemed to lack interest in their child. I met them in an emergency session and after some minutes the husband said he had noticed a small change in his wife. I asked the woman if she also had felt that and she said "Yes, last two days". "How and when exactly did you start to feel like that?" I asked her. She said "When I took the phone and scheduled the session". She continued to describe what was in her mind and what she did before taking the phone – she had to take care of her baby and herself, and she knew her husband supported her.

Goals. They need to be small, achievable, detailed and able to measure as earlier mentioned. The taxi metaphor used by Insoo Kim Berg (personal communication, 1991) is very telling. When you go by taxi the driver asks you where you want to go. He/she doesn't drive you to a place of his/her priorities. The same goes for therapy. It is all about asking the client where he/she is heading and wants to achieve – partly because it is the clients preferred future we are talking about and partly because the necessity to explore and find out what the session needs to focus on. The golf metaphor of Michael Hoyt (2020) – "It will a long day on the golf course if you don't know where the holes are" is another way of describing the importance of knowing where the client is heading.

Many couples attending couple sessions tell the counsellor their problem is communication, and they want to have some tools to enhance their relationship. This is very vaguely expressed and in collaboration you need to figure out what this means in detailed and concrete terms. What parts of their communication does not work? How do they talk to each other? What do they want to do differently? How will they notice the difference when they talk to each other in a way they both appreciate? What specific tools are they asking for? Questions and answers can be varied endlessly, and this is needed to make goal descriptions concrete and detailed.

Alliance/Collaboration is the fourth aspect of brief therapy and consists of many parts. Alliance is an important concept used in many therapeutic models and is often described as a continued process, but we know that first impression occur within a few milli seconds and these often remains for some time (Willis and Todorow, 2006). In brief therapy models the assumption is – *collaboration starts immediately*. Sometimes this is evident directly:

I was interviewing my colleague and the couple she had seen six months ago and before I had the chance to say anything the woman said: "I knew directly from the start that this would be fine and end well". Naturally I asked her how she knew this before they even had begun the session. The woman in details described how my colleague opened the door to the office, greeted them welcome and how she was equally interested in both her and her husband. The ground was laid for collaboration in the session. (Söderquist, 2009b, in Swedish).

The two concepts *follow and lead* are very important in therapeutic sessions. We all know if we are too pushy the client's response might be to resist and if we don´t do enough disappointment will be the reaction from the clients. Therapeutic sessions can be described as a dance in which clients and therapists take turns in following and leading. As therapist it is about following the client but also about challenging him/her in a gentle and respectful way when questioning the client's old habits. Together we find a balance between enough similar and enough different (Andersen, 1991) which the client can recognise but also help create the space for new perspectives and ideas. Anther expression is fit. Client and therapist need to find a way of talking, using the same "language" and to generate a feeling of understanding. This is an act of delicate balancing and sometimes a huge challenge. Harlene Anderson (1997) and Furman and Ahola (1992) use the words guest and host and Michael Hoyt talks about caddie and golf player (2000). All these descriptions aim to emphasise the importance of humble collaboration with clients on their premises.

There are two ways to follow and lead in sessions: echoing and follow up questions. Echoing is to repeat what the client just said which is one way of telling the client you listened to her/him. At the same time, it encourages the client to go on and in more detail describe problems and goals. Follow up and asking more detailed questions is another way of showing the client you are present, are listening and want to hear more from the client. Both therapist behaviours are examples of follow and lead – therapist/counsellor ignores some of the things the client mentioned and can then react and invite the client to describe other things she/he said. To curiously ask more questions sometimes give the client an opportunity to tell things never told before. This is the case of Anna:

Anna had a long history with a hard upbringing and sickness. To try to get a hold of her story and to make it a bit concentrated I asked her to make a diagram of her ups and downs the last ten years. When I asked her what she did when she was in down periods she said: "I met therapists" and when I asked her about her up periods she said: "I met normal people". I couldn´t help laughing and said: "I see myself as both normal and a therapist. How do you want me as therapist to behave to not make it worse for you and how do you want me to behave as a normal person to support you?" This started a very constructive discussion of what kind of help and therapy Anna wanted.

After a year we summarised and evaluated the therapy. Anna said that the best of all with our sessions was; "You never said I was crazy!". I hadn't thought of this but hearing Anna saying this I was reminded of Anna in every session asking me if she was crazy. Every time I answered "I don't know. What you have been telling me could be a sign of what really happened to you or could be your fantasies. I don't know". This had been very important and crucial to Anna and I didn't get it until Anna told me when we were to terminate therapy.

A couple example: The woman scheduled One at a Time (OAAT) counselling and surprised her husband in the session by telling us what went on in her mind before taking the phone. His reaction was "I am glad you told me, I knew you were competent but I was so worried and didn't see your efforts". My questions opened up and made it possible for the wife to tell her husband.

Letting the clients choose and believe he/she can manage more than they know is also collaboration. The task of therapists and counsellors is to make this clear to the clients. As therapists and counsellors we are not so important as we might think. People close to the lives of the clients we see; partners, parents, siblings, children and friends are of most importance before, during and after therapy is terminated.

We met Cilla earlier in the chapter and she told me:

I asked her what kind of advices she would give other girls in her situation having been raped. Cilla summarised: "Live your life normally. Get away from people pitying you. Get help from people supporting you." By living normally Cilla meant doing the things usually being done in spite of being afraid and not letting what had happened rule your life.

Alain Topor (2001) presents results from interviews in his book *Återhämtning från svåra psykiska störningar* (in English: *Recovery from severe mental disorders*) which has been important to me through the years. Two of the things that patients reported were crucial to me and I have tried to bear this in mind in my sessions with couples. Some patients reported they could go on all day long planning to put on their shoes intending to get some coffee in the kitchen. They fought hard and it was exhausting. The staff often did not see this at all, they saw a catatonic patient sitting in the same position all day. For those patients it was crucial when the staff noticed these small and tiny steps of recovering. Years later they reported in follow up interviews this was what helped them recover. Another important thing the patients reported as crucial for their recovery was when the therapist "broke a therapeutic rule" – behaved a little bit unusually and not agreed upon from the start. These small therapeutic behaviours could be – prolonging the session with a few minutes or suggesting the sessions be a walk and talk session in the park. For the patients this was the confirmation for them that the therapist saw, heard, understood and cared about them as human beings.

This told me the importance of noticing and affirming even the smallest behaviour, work, effort, fighting and personal agency. It also points out the importance of therapist being willing and prepared to "break some therapeutic rules" to show the clients they are more important than therapeutic models and conventions.

Ann and Tom was a couple in their forties with two small children. Ann had delusions, heard voices and was hospitalised. Her psychiatrist asked me to do a consultation interview and Ann accepted this arrangement. This was later followed by several consultations on Anns initiative. She told me and her husband two things in the consultation interviews that is still vivid in my memory: 1. When I asked her if I could talk to her voices she said "They won't talk to you", and I said "Will they hear me?" "Yes they will ", she said and gave permission. I talked to her voices for a while mainly about the concern for Ann and her wellbeing. She later reported that the day after the interview was a miracle day. 2. Ann also described how she when the voices forced her to throw things at people did this but carefully avoided to hit people. She resisted the voices and were responsible in very difficult and strange situations.

Is SST/OAAT breaking traditional therapeutic rules, adapting to the needs and doings of some clients or is SST/OAAT something quite new? Before focusing these questions let us talk about therapeutic questioning.

Therapeutic questioning

In the 1980s Karl Tomm presented his model of therapeutic questions – lineal, circular, reflexive and strategic (Tomm, 1987; 1988).

Tomm's categorising and definitions of therapeutic questioning were important to therapists in the 1980s and 1990s. Vertically linear and circular assumptions and horizontally orienting and strategic intentions made the differences between therapeutic models very clear. Lineal and strategic questions build on linear assumptions and are characteristic of traditional, objective or empirical paradigms. These questions are inquiring and their purpose are to understand the family system. Circular and reflexive questions build on circular assumptions and are characteristic of systemic or social constructionistic paradigms. These questions aim for facilitating changes in the family system. Examples of questions (Tomm, 1987; 1988):

- *Lineal*: Direct questions focused on how something was done. Who did what when and how?
- *Circular*: How come we meet today? Who is most worried? Who is least worried? What is your father doing when you and your mother talk?

- *Reflexive*: If there was anything not clarified between you who would be the first to apologise? When you/her/him have found a way to take care who will be the first to notice?
- *Strategic*: Do you notice/how do you notice your wife being disappointed when you withdraw? When will you take responsibility for your own life?

Later Karl Tomm together with Carsten Hornstrup and Johansen developed and revised the model. Time was included as an important dimension (horisontal) and vertically constructing and clarifying replaced assumptions. The names of the questions were changed and the concept *co-* was introduced to point out the joint action of collaboration (Hornstrup, Tomm and Johansen, 2009).

Examples of questions in the revised model:

- *Situating questions*: What are you most worried about at the moment? How do you look at what is happening right now? Please tell me what you are experiencing as most problematic right now?
- *Perspectives questions*: How would your best friend describe your situation at the moment? How would the person knowing you very well describe your strengths?
- *Possibilities questions*: What would be the best result of this session? What are your best hopes for this session? Imagine you reach this tomorrow what will be the first sign you notice?
- *Initiatives questions*: What can you do to go in the directions of your goals? From what we have been talking about what do you see as possible to make happen right now?

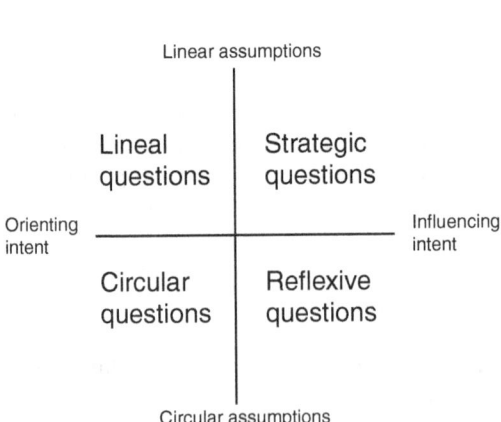

The Original Model 1988

Figure 6.1 Karl Tomm's original model. Power Point presentation in Sweden 2017 and 2019

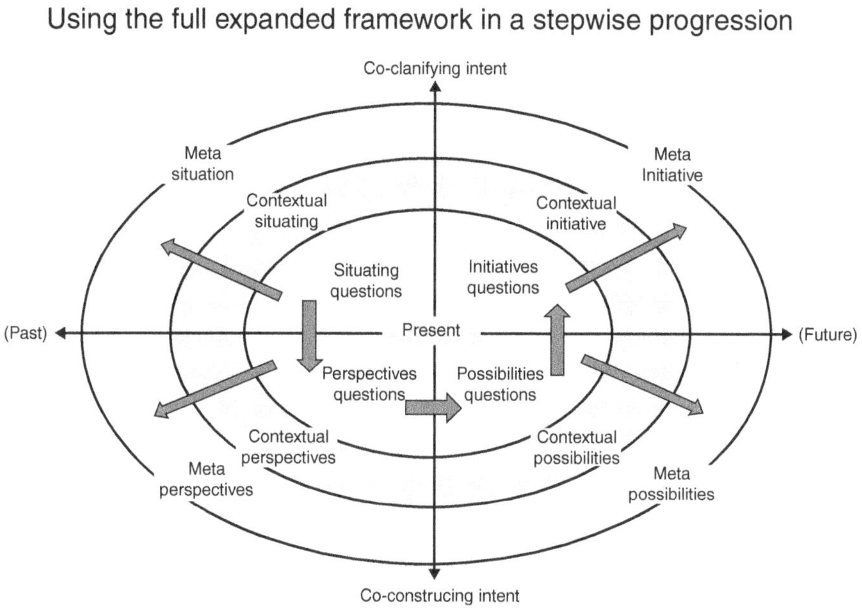

Using the full expanded framework in a stepwise progression

Figure 6.2 Karl Tomm's revised model for interventive interviewing (Hornstrup, Tomm and Johansen, 2009)

Hornstrup, Tomm and Johansen (2009) also expand the model by contextual and meta questions to a wider context and to a meta perspective.

Examples of contextual questions: If you were in another culture or institutional context how would your situation/problem been looked at? What institutional changes can you imagine helping you move forward? (relational possibility question)? If you were to act upon your plans how would your reputation change?

Examples of meta questions: What additional questions can I use to help me understand your situation? (contextual meta-perspective question). Who else can I ask who maybe look at your situation a bit different? (perspective meta question). Are there any more questions I can ask you that might help you go outside the box? (possibility meta question).

Hornstrup, Tomm and Johansen's categorising and classifying of how questions in therapy can be used in other contexts is very interesting. The model can be a questions library or a reference book to therapists and consultants when doing their best to make sessions and consultations varied and helpful to clients. It is not possible here to do their model justice, and I refer to Hornstrup, Tomm and Johansen (2009).

In our OAAT sessions with couples we often use a question like this: "How will your partner/children/the person who knows you very well notice tomorrow/this weekend/next week the changes you talk about/things going in the right direction/you are co-operating the way you want it to be/you are having a good time?"

Tomm see these questions as *relational context initiative questions* – "the question invites the persons to stretch their imagination beyond their own change possibilities and how the change would be noticed by significant others is a way to stabilise proposed changes. The questions also draw upon a person's preferred reputation in the minds of others which could add to their motivation to follow through" (Tomm, personal communication, 2019). Questions like these have many functions in sessions, can be constructive and give a lot of new ideas.

In long-term therapy and series of counselling sessions, contextual questions (to clarify the client's situation) are used, followed by perspective questions (to clarify and make descriptions deeper) and possibility questions (to describe new possibilities). Later in sessions, initiative questions are used to prepare the clients work on their own after therapy to change their lives/reach their goals.

OAAT therapists do all these things in one session, focus on what is most important today to the client/couple and investigate and describe this by means of possibility and initiative questions.

Chapter 7

Sources of Inspiration

Martin Söderquist

Since my colleagues and I first began to work with Single Session Therapy (SST) we have been inspired by the work of many international colleagues. This chapter is a brief summary of these sources of inspiration:

Single Session Therapy, Single Session Walk-in, Single Session Work and Single Session Walk-in Agencies

Session Formats

Single session therapy. Like so many other phenomena, SST began by coincidence. Moshe Talmon worked at Kaiser Permanente Medical Centre in the 1980s and, going through filed records, he discovered a large proportion of the clients attended only one session, regardless of the therapeutic orientation of the therapists. After initial follow-up, retrospective study of clinical charts and follow-up phone calls Talmon, Bob Rosenbaum and Michael Hoyt together did a first prospective study. Of those who participated in SST, 58% elected to complete in one session, even though more sessions were available.

This led to the start of a research project together with his colleagues Hoyt and Rosenbaum to find a model for maximising the first and often the only session a client had with a therapist. The experiences from this project were summarised in *Single Session Therapy* (Talmon, 1990). SST builds on the assumption that the clients have the potential to activate their resources to spontaneous healing and problem solving, on their own or together with their networks of family and friends. The processes of changes are present all the time, and when the clients decide to reach out for a therapist, they have already made a giant step. In Talmon's model, three parts are integrated to a whole: (1) intake procedure/telephone call a week before session, (2) session, (3) follow-up by telephone. In this model the session is planned and scheduled in advance and the clients are sometimes given a task: "Please notice what is going on that you want to continue" (de Shazer, 1988; 1991) before the session. In a way, Talmon, Hoyt and Rosenbaum's SST model consists of three contacts between client and therapist but only one face-to-face meeting (Rosenbaum et al., 1990; Hoyt et al., 1992).

DOI: 10.4324/9781003305774-7

Single Session Walk-in. Inspired by Talmon and as way to reduce waiting lists and increase accessibility, Eastside Family Centre in Calgary, Canada began offering single session therapy beginning 1990'(Slive et al., 1995). Nancy McElheran and Arnie Slive were two of the initiative taking therapists. The centre chose walk-in as a suitable format. The clients did not have to schedule in advance; they could just show up in the reception. No intake procedure, no before-hand information and no planned follow up. A service with low thresholds and maximum accessibility and service was created. Follow ups showed very good results (see Appendix). No client had to wait more than 20 minutes until they were in the session with the therapist and his/her team. The clients were given an information sheet and were asked to answer a few questions (problems, hopes for the session) for filing records and documentation. If in cases of being in the wrong place or if the clients have more urgent needs the therapist joins (sometimes called a "warm hand-off") the client on a visit to a more suitable clinic instead of making referrals on the phone or on paper. The walk-in service is open six days a week and can offer varied help to clients. There are always full-time therapists, interested colleagues and intern trainees led by a shift coordinator coordinating the team. The walk-in service sees three to ten clients a day and a total of 3,500 clients a year.

A similar service is Reach Out Centre for Kids (ROCK) in Toronto, Canada. They can be found in five different locations in Ontario. The follow ups and evaluations being done show 50 % of their clients (approximately 2,000 clients a year) report one session is enough, and the others report they need additional sessions. ROCKS conclusions are the clients know when they need help, they have the knowledge and resources and their contexts are crucial. (Harper-Jacques et al., 2008, Harper-Jacques et al., 2014).

Karen Young and her colleagues in Ontario have proceeded in building up walk-in services and nowadays there are more than 100 services in Ontario (Young, 2018. in Hoyt et al., 2018). Organisations like *Mental Health Centres, Family Health Centres and Canadian Mental Health Association* run these walk-in services. They are not always called walk-in instead called *Talk-in clinic, Session at a time service and What's up clinic.* Some of these services do 10–20 minutes screening interviews before the session and the team prepare the session with a pre session team discussion. Other services like Eastside Family Centre Walk-In service just asks the clients to fill in some forms before the session (Hoyt et al., 2018).

Single Session Work. Bouverie Centre, Victoria Family Institute in Melbourne, Australia was inspired by Talmon's model in the early 1990s. They chose to use the original model with intake procedure, task, session and follow up. The centre names their format Single Session Work (SSW) since the centre doesn't regard the format as therapy or consultation. They see it as a service offer to the clients. SST implies short waiting list, easy access and every therapist's assumption that every session can be the last (as if the session is the last). At the same time, it is important and characteristic for SSW that the door is always open for another SSW session or other forms of planned and continued sessions. The goal is to optimise the possibilities of the session by letting the clients guide the therapist and by focusing the small changes that can be made. All clients and families are offered a first session with two therapists and before session a letter with questions is sent to the client/family to be brought to the session. In the telephone follow up some weeks after the SSW session the clients/families and the therapist collaboratively decide: more sessions, referral to another service or clinic, one more SSW session or "Are we done?".

The therapists at Eastside Family Centre, ROCK and Bouverire are pragmatic and inspired by several different models of therapy like Solution Focused Brief therapy, Narrative Therapy, Family Therapy and Cognitive Behavioural Therapy (CBT). Most important is the fit for clients and how useful the sessions are. To know that one size does not fit all is also important.

Bouverie Centre has by extended training programs created a centre with different teams and specialities. The centre has also for many years implemented single session work in the state of Victoria. As a a curiosity it can be mentioned that Jeff Young, director of Bouverie, has developed a way of working with reluctant and unmotivated clients he calls "no bullshit therapy" (Young, personal communication, 2014).

Single Session Walk-in-Clinics. Arnie Slive was one of the therapists developing SST and walk-in in Canada. Later on he moved back to USA where he collaborated with Monte Bobele in starting up walk-in clinics in Austin and San Antonio (Slive and Bobele, 2011,). In their book *When one hour is all you have* they describe in detail how to do walk-in and how this is done in other clinics around the world. The model for training Slive and Bobele has introduced in Texas – an experienced therapist and six trainees work as a team; one trainee in the session room and the rest of the team in another room in front of the tv-screen – has proven the effectiveness of the model. All clients are offered a walk-in session or a scheduled session and they are informed many clients report one session is enough but the possibility of more sessions is available.

SST Literature Overview. The ground-breaking work of Talmon, Hoyt and Rosenbaum's and Talmon's book *Single Session Therapy (*1990) inspired several organisations and agencies to implement and develop different formats of SST. This process continued by follow ups and research and now SST is going global. Three international conferences (2012, 2015 and 2019) followed by three books summarising the state of art (Hoyt et al.,2014, 2018, 2021) and in addition several articles and books have contributed to growing interest and knowledge amongst therapists and counsellors.

This brief overview (for a fuller overview, see the books mentioned above) will concentrate on implementation of SST, SST in several contexts and integration of SST and therapeutic models.

Implementation of SST mindset. Eastside Family Centre, Canada, Bouverie Centre, Australia and Our Lady of the Lake University, USA have been the main centres and hubs in the development of different SST formats, inspiration and implementation of SST in other organisations and in other countries. Implementation of SST in Australia has been written about by Jeff Young and his colleagues (Young et al., 2012) pointing to what is important to consider when introducing new mind sets and practices and how this can be done. Arnie Slive and Monte Bobeles book *When one hour is all you have* (2011) answers many questions about Walk-in and describes the work being done by different agencies in Canada and the USA.

Karen Young in Canada writes about the rapid growth of Walk-in clinics in Ontario (Young, 2018). Flavio Cannistrà and Piccirilli (2018) in Italy describe the Italian version of SST which is growing strongly in Italy.

It is not an easy task to implement something new; existing misunderstandings, resistance from colleagues and the necessary support (or lack of) from managers are real challenges for those trying. Different ways to do this is described by Renkin, Alexander and Wyder; McDonald, Hickey, Wyder; and McElheran (in Hoyt et al., 2021).

In Sweden our work in Malmö has inspired other couple counselling teams to start offering OAAT to couples in their communities.

SST in different contexts. The SST mind set is fit in many contexts and can be applied in many organisations and agencies. Mental Health Settings, Family and Youth Centres and Counselling Agencies, some of them with waiting lists, have found SST very useful (see Hoyt et al., 2021). Agencies and centres working with individual clients in Australia has been inspired by the Bouverie model for briefly engaging and inclusion of families in the treatment and care of the client, The model, Single Session Family Counselling, is described by Brendan O´Hanlon and Naomi Rotten (in Hoyt et al., 2021).

Pam Rycroft describes how to capture the moment in supervision and Sandy Harper-Jacques presents how to structure supervision with a group of skilled therapists (in Hoyt et al., 2018). Windy Dryden combines lectures and consultations with predominantly professionals attending in London (in Hoyt et al., 2021). Harper-Jacques and Houger-Limacher emphasise the contextual sensitivity as a cornerstone of supervision (2009).

When disasters and catastrophes hit people there is usually no time, no possibilities and not a chance to engage them in ongoing trauma treatment. There is only one meeting or one brief session available. SST mind set and practice is well fit in these circumstances. Miller (in Slive and Bobele, 2011) points out strategies for disaster mental health counselling doing single session intervention after the wake of Hurricane Katrina and Rafale Nunez and Jorge Abia use Eriksonian Strategic Hypnotherapy for disasters in Mexico (in Hoyt et al. 2021).

Literature on therapy and counselling is most often written by and for the western society therapists with its dominating narrative of a medical mind set and long-term ongoing therapy/problem solving. Non-Western societies are culturally very different and John Miller, working in Cambodja and China has in three chapters in Hoyt et al. (2014; 2018; 2021) described how SST mindset and practice can be introduced in these countries. Miller describes the cultural and contextual sensitive approach and the willingness to do things the Asian way, involving mobile teams in very remote places, instead of counselling the way we in Western societies are trained in. (in Hoyt et al., 2018; 2021).

SST mind set can be a perfect fit when coming to service and counselling in remote places and in indigenous communities. Sophia Sorensen (Canada) gives us her story of counselling far away from the agency office and with a humble will to connect with leadership in the indigenous community and Alison Elliott, James Dokona and Henry von Doussa (Australia) point out the decolonising, hope installing, trust-building aspects of SST that appears to be a fit to Indigenous families in their communities (in Hoyt et al., 2021).

There are very few, or none at all, mentioning of SST and Couples counselling and since the Malmö Couple Counselling is specialised in couple relationships and exclusively working with couple counselling we have for many years developed OAAT with Couples and gained important experiences (Söderquist, 2018; Söderquist et al., 2021.)

Integration of SST and therapeutic models. All SST formats like SSW, Walk-in and OAAT are based on the principles of SST and most practitioners integrate these principals with their own preferred therapeutic models. All kinds of brief therapy models fit with SST and are applied in many contexts. Eastside Family Centre work systemically, and their teamwork uses the five-phase model originated in The Milan Model (Selvini Palazzoli, 1978). Karen Young (2017) and her Canadian colleagues integrate SST mind set with narrative approaches. South Calgary Health (Harper-Jacques et al., 2008) and Windy Dryden (2019) integrate SST and CBT. Windy Dryden also integrates *SST and Rational Emotive Behavior* (2020).

Solution-Focused Brief Therapy, the model I and my OAAT colleagues see as a good fit and preferable when doing OAAT sessions with couples, is mentioned in many articles and books. To give a few examples: George, Iveson and Ratner (1999), McElheran et al. (2014) and Robinson, Harvey, McDonald and Honegger (2021). This model emphasises focusing on strengths and competencies, client goals and is client driven.

The development of SST formats in different contexts has formed a lot of guidelines and practices which is too far to go into here. Paul and van Ommeren (2013) is an excellent example and Hoyt et al.'s three books (Hoyt et al., 2015; 2018; 2021) contains several descriptions of guidelines and practices.

Brief Stories: How We Were Inspired[1]

There are many different roads to Rome, as the saying goes, and there are many ways for couple counsellors to make the leap to an OAAT mindset. It is impossible to describe them all but inspired by the collection *Therapist Stories of Inspiration, Passion, and Renewal: What's Love Got to Do with It?* (Hoyt, 2013) we want to share some stories of our own. We all had a head start – we were already trained in family and brief therapy.

MARTIN SÖDERQUIST: When I first read Talmon's book in the beginning of the 1990s I was thrilled and excited. In a way, it was a perfect fit – I and my colleagues already worked in a family-oriented and solution- focused way. I wanted to implement Single Session Therapy immediately. This wasn´t possible for many reasons and it wasn't until I began working as a couple counsellor in the beginning of the 2000s that I really could start planning SST/OAAT.

What finally got me going was a telephone follow-up that we did with 68 unplanned single session couples. Many couples told us "one session was enough." Some of the couples reported that "we had decided to attend one session" – but they didn´t tell the counsellor. I realized that some couples asked – not always in a direct manner – for one session and not more. This reminded me of how important it is to offer clients what they want and when they ask for it instead of making clients fit into your preferred therapy model or the administration of the organisation.

This was my leap more than ten years ago and for me, there is no way back.

KARIN WULFF: Paradoxically, it´s been a long and slow process for me to embrace brief OAAT. Trained in solution-focused theory and after a decade of daily Solution Focused Brief Therapy sessions with individuals one might think it would be easy. It was trickier than I expected.

I started implementing the mindset of OAAT in 2015, in the context of couple counselling. Hard work and a lot of practice made me overcome the challenging parts and enjoy the energy and possibilities in each session.

To me it's a question about timing. Timing in several aspects: if a client can get help when they need it, you offer the right question, affirmation and intervention in the right moment of the session. I find it slightly more challenging to work with couples compared to individuals. Practicing OAAT I've become more disciplined with focus and timing, which I also find helpful in other forms of clinical work.

It´s a privilege to work in a context that offers counselling when people ask for it. My readiness to be there when a couple is looking for change is something to aim for in every session.

A lot of things can change if your timing is good.

LARS DANNERUP: How do we know if things we talked about were useful? How do we know anything about the future? How do we know if change happens quickly or slowly? The simple answer to that is, we don't know it until after it has happened. That means that we can only do our best in the single moment.

At the beginning of my career as a therapist I had the good fortune to be a member of a team which on several occasions was trained and supervised by Steve de Shazer and Insoo Kim Berg. Especially two things made a huge impact on me. One thing to remember is that "every session could be the last session" and another thing is to always "ask the client where they want to go, don't get started until you know their destination."

Many years ago a woman in her late twenties stepped into my office. The only thing I knew about her was that she had been a heroin addict since the age of 13 and been in and out of treatment since then. It would have been easy to think that one session couldn't possibly make a difference. And, of course, I did. With de Shazer and Insoo Berg in mind, I just started out with where she wanted to go and some minutes into the session I asked the Miracle Question. She started by saying: "I'll get up in the morning, have a cup of coffee and then I'll be off to work." The session continued with us exploring her thoughts and feelings regarding the work she had pictured herself doing.

I meet her on and off in the community. She's now a teacher in a high school. Once she told me it was that one session that made the miracle.

Thirty years down the road it still can be hard work, but through her help and many many others I now understand how helpful one single session can be.

MALENA CRONHOLM-NOUICER: Therapists still don't know very much about how change happens. What we know is that life is constantly in motion whether we wish or not. For me, OAAT makes it a possibility to collaboratively create with the couple a space for hopes of relational movement. Sometimes this can be an intensive deep dive into something important for the couple, or a careful dipping of a toe in the water.

I work with OAAT convinced that one single session can make a difference. My experience is that OAAT requires curiosity and careful attention to capture the first glimpse of what a move in the right direction could be or how a small change could ripple for the couple.

I will never forget the man who spontaneously said after the session: "Good God, what a relief! I thought you [his partner] were going to end our relationship in this session." Together we noted and realized that, on the contrary, the session was focused on the couple's desire for closeness. The session had given them more hope of such a possibility.

Note

1 This part of the chapter is published in Söderquist et al., 2021

Chapter 8

Frequently Asked Questions about OOAT

Martin Söderquist

Over the years the couple counselling team in Malmö has worked with Single Session Therapy (SST) and (since 2016) with One at a Time (OAAT), and we have received a lot of questions from couples we have seen and from our colleagues. The questions have arisen from interest and curiosity, but they have also been critical and doubtful. This has forced us to rethink, reflect and define what we are doing in collaboration with the couples we see. This has been necessary in order to develop our methods and our way of conducting sessions.

In the following pages I will go through some of the questions we have faced. The aim is to clarify what OAAT is not and then go on clarifying what OAAT is as we see it.

Isn't OAAT a new model of therapy? All therapists and counsellors, regardless of their preferred therapy model, most often meet client for only one session.

Single session therapy, walk-in and OAAT are session formats for clients choosing one or few sessions with therapists and counsellors. In a way these formats resemble what is called consultation: A client and therapist agreement on one session. The client has maybe seen a doctor or a psychologist and she/he wants a consultation or a "second opinion". The therapist might ask for a consultation together with his/her client in order to get new perspectives to proceed in therapy. Consultation interviews and OAAT can be conducted by therapists and counsellors with different and varied theoretical and practical orientations. OAAT is not associated to a special model of therapy.

Isn't OAAT a kind of light version of real therapy? A whole therapy is not possible in one session, and "ten sessions in one" is not possible. But it is possible to achieve a lot in one session enough for clients to continue what they need to do at home. Therapy is not needed for everyone - most people solve their problems on their own and sometimes all what is needed is confirmation they are on the right track or they are "normal". OAAT might not be therapy, but the session can be therapeutic (Young and Jebreen, 2020; Francis and Clarkin, 1981).

What is the evidence for OAAT? Considering the fact these session formats haven´t existed for more than a couple of years the time has been too short to

DOI: 10.4324/9781003305774-8

allow Randomised Controlled Trials (RCT) studies. There has only been one RCT study made so far, by Perkins (2006) in Australia. Nowadays we do not talk about evidence-based models; we talk about evidence-based practice, which is a combination of the following: evaluation of models, the clients' experiences and the therapist's experiences. This definition of evidence-based practice includes SST, Walk-in and OAAT (see Appendix).

Isn't it necessary to make assessments before therapy and consultations? From a medical point of view, assessments must be made before treatment begins. Daryl Chow (2018) calls this the *intake model* and this model according to Chow results in drop-outs and briefer therapies than the clients need. The *engagement model* in which the therapist listens to what the client wants and wishes stands in contrast to the *intake model*. The aim here is to help the client having a positive and constructive experience in the first session. It is important the client get something out of the session. Chow talks a lot about drop out and the importance of longer therapies (he claims he has prolonged the therapies since he started doing engagement therapy). It gives me the idea the *engagement model* is a way of keeping clients in therapy and avoid drop-outs. OAAT represents a different stance. I will come back to this in more detail.

In systems theory and collaborative models planning and structuring sessions are joint and collaborative. If clients are seen as their own experts, there is no problem, and it follows naturally that the clients know what are best for them. They are able to decide what is good for them, what kind of sessions they want, how many sessions they are willing to attend and attend outpatient treatment and voluntary sessions by their own choice. Seen this way the therapist/counsellor is the expert on conducting sessions and the client is the expert on her/himself. In my book *Delaktighet* (Participation in English, Söderquist& Suskin-Holmqvist, 2006, in Swedish) we present thinking and practice in regard to involontary and compulsory assessments. Different models for assessments and evaluations are presented with examples from Child Protection Service and Child and Adolescent Psychiatry.

Isn't more than an hour needed to create an alliance? First impressions are immediately as mentioned earlier but it may take more or less time to gain the clients' confidence and create an alliance. Common factor research (Hubble, Duncan and Miller, 1999; Wampold, 2001; Wampold and Imel, 2015) show us the importance of therapist-client relationship and that alliance takes some time to create. But we also know that the allotted time that we have decides how we structure and utilise the time we have. If we only have a brief amount of time we must focus on the most important and drop the rest. It is possible to create an alliance very rapid. OAAT has proven that (Young and Jebreen, 2020).

Is OAAT suitable for all clients? No, definitely not. Many clients, couples and families want several sessions - they think their problems can't be handled in one session. Or they think their problems are too serious and longer therapy is needed. Of course, they must be offered this. Couple Counselling Team in Malmö offer all couples what we call Traditional Counselling – possibility to see the same counsellor for several sessions over time. We also offer one to three sessions – the same counsellor for a restricted number of sessions. We do not decide what session format the couples need; it is up to the couples to choose. In advance, we know their names, age and if and how many children they have. We see all couples scheduling appointments, and if they need anything else than counselling sessions, we help them to the right team or clinic. For us the only exception is couples in child custody and access fights. They are referred to a special team in Malmö.

Is OAAT a problem-solver for all problems? From what has been said previously on quantitative and qualitative changes (first and second order changes) problems can be solved in unexpected, surprising and odd ways. Eastside Family Centre, Bouverie Centre and SST work in various areas of catastrophes (Hoyt et al., 2018; Hoyt, Young and Rycroft, 2021) have shown the usefulness of SST, Walk-in and OAAT in many very difficult contexts. By this, we do not mean that all victims of torture, clients with psychosis diagnoses or dangerous intimate partner violence couples can solve their problems in one session. These clients can benefit from one session if they have the session in the right time, when they need it, get the strength to do the changes they might have to do or come to the conclusion they do not want to schedule therapy or consultation. The OAAT session can lay the ground for the clients constructive moving forward.

Is OAAT fit for all spheres of activities? The short answer is – OAAT does not suit every situation. For Child Protection workers, Probation officers or clinics and teams ruled by strict laws it is hard or impossible to use OAAT. Outpatient teams in different clinics and centres have more varied possibilities regardless of what problems clients have. OAAT as the first and sometimes the only session is an option, and after the session the clients decide how to continue.

If the clients want additional sessions – are they only offered one session? When we began with single session therapy we often heard expressions like "Only one session?", "Can´t you have more?" and "Is this really true?". When following up we saw 20% of those choosing single session therapy requested additional sessions and that was not a problem for us. After a few years we called our work OAAT to clarify the agreement was one session, but the clients were free to return. Nowadays we are careful to clarify the couples are entitled to choose traditional counselling if they need or want additional sessions.

The concept SST can be misleading. On one occasion a man called me and wanted to schedule a single session and I asked as I usually do: "Who will join you?", and the guy briefly said: "I will come alone – it is single session". We did find out the slight misunderstanding (but of course he could come to session alone) and scheduled the session. Later we changed from single session to OAAT.

Isn´t it really morally right and ethical to offer the couples the same counsellor if they return for additional sessions? We clearly inform the couples we can´t promise they can see the same counsellor if they return for additional sessions, but they have the possibility to request this when they schedule second or third session. We try to meet them in this if it is possible. Eastside Family Centre´s experiences are – clients schedule an appointment with the centre, not with a specified therapist. (McElheran et al., 2014; McElheran, personal communication, 2015). The centre is more important than the person. To see the same therapist if you return for additional sessions can be important to the couples, as they do not have to start from the beginning again every session. This applies to individual clients too. For our part, we point out to the couples that we do not start from the beginning. We collaboratively go through what the couple made of the last session and what they have been doing until today. The couple does not have to tell their full background or whole story.

Isn´t single session therapy, walk-in and OAAT just a tool to save the economy of the community, to cut budgets and make waiting lists shorter? It is true many centres in Canada and USA began as projects to make waiting lists shorter. In many cases it turned out to work like that. For us in Malmö it has never been the case and our waiting list hasn´t been shortened. We have had an ever-increasing number of couples scheduling appointments.

Is OAAT special? OAAT is both special and very ordinary. There are no huge differences between OAAT and a first session of a longer therapy. When we began single session therapy our group, together with colleagues not working with single session therapy regularly watched video-taped sessions and compared single session therapy with ordinary first sessions. We had difficulties seeing the differences. What was different in single session therapy was; more directness and a greater focus and concentration on the clients desired and wanted goals in the nearest future. If you see the single session as the only session available, you need to think and do a little bit different than you are trained in other therapy models but it requires a huge leap in thinking and practice.

Chapter 9

OAAT Mindset – Thinking and Practice

Martin Söderquist

"Although brief relational work is now accepted, going from brief to OAAT relational work, beginning in the 1990–2000s, was another giant leap. Going from thinking in processes/serial thinking to one off sessions in OAAT is a great challenge."

(Söderquist et al., 2021)

One at a Time (OAAT) counselling is not a fit for all therapists and counsellors. To work in the spirit of OAAT requires many considerations, a meta perspective on therapy and a way of thinking and doing that is new and maybe overwhelming.

You need to believe in the competence of the clients and the fact that the therapist is not superior expert. This kind of thinking and doing is necessary. It is not the therapy model that is crucial.

Generally speaking, all therapists and counsellors do a great job when they use the therapy model they believe in and which fits them.

Thinking and Practice

In English and international literature, the concept *Mindset* is used to describe the thinking and doing in therapy or counselling. In all therapy being done we are influenced by our training and personal preferences. Our mindsets include many presuppositions within our language. When we ask the client; "What are you hoping for?" our suppositions are that the clients have hopes. If we ask, "Why are we sitting here today?", we suppose in the same way there is a real reason. Presuppositions are sometimes conscious and expressed, sometimes not so thoroughly considered but they are present all the time. Suppositions are not true, right or evidence based but OAAT thinking and doing suppositions are defining the session format.

I break up the thinking/doing/presuppositions in: Generally, resources and competencies, goals and collaboration.

DOI: 10.4324/9781003305774-9

General Aspects

- Problems can be solved in a variety of ways
- The OAAT session is all that is planned – clients and couples can return for additional sessions when/if they wish. It is their decision.
- The session is a complete whole
- Every session is a new one. If the couple return their situation is new and the session is a new one
- Expectancies of change and progress today/tomorrow – not in the future
- OAAT is not a part of a special therapy model but builds on ideas from competence and brief therapy models. The OAAT session adapts to the needs and wishes of the clients not expecting the couple to adapt to the therapy model.
- OAAT doesn´t fit all – one size does not fit all, as the saying goes. Neither clients nor therapists
- Therapy according to Steve de Shazer is reminding the client where they are heading and how to continue in that direction (de Shazer, personal communication, 1993)

Resources and Competencies

- The strengths and competencies of the client/couple/family are the most important factors to explain positive outcomes from therapy
- Before the session the couple has tried to solve their problems and made some progress in their lives – pre session change (de Shazer, 1991)
- People are not isolated islands they have persons in their network supporting and helping them
- Clients/couples/families have ideas and plans, and "you don´t have to cross the river to get to the water"

Goals

- The most important goal is what the clients express – not what the therapist thinks
- The goals need to be small, realistic, be the start of something and which can be continued when it works
- A goal for OAAT is to aim for, when ending session or at follow up, clients saying they have one or several ideas how to manage their situation or problems ("To know my way about") or express hope what can be achieved in the future

Collaboration

- Therapists need to meet the client where they are in their minds and contexts

- Therapists ought to follow the clients by careful listening and continued asking of what the clients express as important to them
- Therapists ought to strive to work in the direction of the goals the clients have expressed
- Therapists ought to focus here and now and keep it simple
- The task of the therapist is not to use the session to motivate, prepare or lay the ground for next session or prolonged therapy. This is the crucial difference in the comparison with Chows *engagement model*
- In OAAT one session is planned and all involved do their best to make the session beneficial and useful to the clients
- Therapists ought to use their own preferred model and way of conducting sessions
- Therapists need to be humble – therapists are caddies to the golf player/ clients (Hoyt, 2000; 2017)

There are differences in models when looking at therapy sessions. Solution focused brief therapy sees every session as a potentially last session. Single session therapy is a client-therapist agreement of one session. Walk-in is a format where the couple come to session when it fits the partners, without intake procedures and having to schedule the session. OAAT with couples is a format where couple and therapist agree upon one session with possibility to return for one or two more sessions scheduled one week ahead.

In the following brief story, a remarkable exercise is described showing the difficulties to really listen and how important this is.

Many years ago I attended a conference, and Steve de Shazer did a plenary seminar. Approximately 250 people were present, and we were all very excited. I was very surprised when I entered the room and Steve who wasn´t known to be very social was standing in the doorway greeting everyone and handshaking. He told us all to grab a paper from one of the three piles. I usually don´t like yellow but for some reason I chose a yellow paper.

Steve began the seminar by asking all with green paper (about 80 people) to leave the room. Some of them protested, but Steve told them he was coming to them in a short while. After they left the room, Steve asked the rest of us to sit in groups of three; the greens were to tell the red and yellow person a story important and significant to her/him, the yellow were to observe and the red were to listen to the story of the green without saying anything. The reds were allowed to nod, move the body and hum and haw. They were not allowed to use words. The reds were also given one more task: they were to pretend listening nonverbally but in reality they were to count all the words in the story of the green were there was the letter T. It is not hard to imagine what happened in the groups of three. The reds had severe difficulties to do both tasks: some of them switched back and forth, some of them did one of the tasks and not the other and some gave up. Some of the greens got furious and stopped their story or tried to tell his/her story to the yellow. Some wanted to discuss with the red "what the f... he/she was doing" and why.

This exercise caused uproar but showed very convincingly the difficulties of the art of listening 100% if we simultaneously have our own ideas and thoughts. It is very hard to really listen if we also have ideas like: "We can talk about this next session", "How will I get the client to see this?" and "What intervention from what therapeutic model can I use here?". The balance of listening to the client and question and reflecting in an affirming way to move forward in the session is the challenge in all therapeutic and counselling sessions.

Creativity and Improvisation

Therapeutic models and guidelines are necessary for everyone doing therapy and counselling. You need a map to know how to conduct the session and in which direction to go. Like all therapeutic models and guidelines, the structure of an OAAT session is valuable to have in mind but is not intended to be forced upon the couple. To follow the lead of the couple requires a lot: not relying too much on your preferred therapeutic model but being sensitive with a toolbox of questions and interventions and most of all open to the possibilities for creativity and improvisation. Couples turn up at the session room for many reasons and with different goals and hopes. In OAAT with couples it is very important to listen to the couple, to follow their lead and at the same time collaboratively create a situation where creativity, playfulness and improvisation can help the couple find new ideas and new behaviour. It is necessary to combine a structure (a map, a thinking and practice) with flexibility and creativity and that is a real challenge.

This reminds me of an interview on television many years ago. Hans Alfredsson (1931–2017), a famous Swedish actor, author and film director was interviewed when he was 70 years old. The journalist asked him what the secret was in how to get that old. Hans answered "The main point is to keep the 11-year-old child within you".

Creativity. When you read about people like Einstein, Nobel prize winners, artists, authors and founders of different therapeutic models it is very easy to think" Where do they get their ideas from – did they have it from the beginning or….?" The debate on creativity as innate, genetic, as a personal trait or something learned in social contexts is ongoing like other debates, such as "Are people evil from the start, or are they evil due to childhood experiences?"

Therapists and counsellors in general are advocates for seeing creativity as learned and developed in social relationships. They believe in and trust the positive and creative forces of human beings and see the possibilities in familial and therapeutic situations.

A lot has been written about creativity, and here I can be brief. According to Wikipedia, the possibility for creative responses exists when knowledge of some facts or themes, as well as knowledge of the creative process and with an inner motivation, come together. Creativity consists of being original, bringing forth new ideas, putting them in action and working them through. Fantasy is a cognitive process while creativity leads to a result.

Jim Wilson discusses in his book *Creativity in times of constraint. A practitioner's companion in mental health and social care* (Wilson, 2018) how creativity, seeing things from another perspective and being outside the box is very important to make possible changes and challenge the constraints forced upon us all by organisations, rules and politics. Jim Wilson is a true advocate for the importance of being open, flexible, curious, unpredictable, humorous, thinking in a different or contradictory way compared to the common or usual way when seeing clients and families. Creativity is a collaborative process.

Improvisation is often described as an activity of making or doing something not planned beforehand. To improvise is to be spontaneous, do things without a manuscript and not follow predestined roads or guidelines. When couples come to therapy they are often nervous, do not know what to expect and most of all they want something beneficial to them to happen in the session. If they meet a therapist who is interested only in assessment and 20 questions about their problems, they might get a little bit frustrated. If the therapist can listen to them, follow their lead and add a little bit of improvising, humour and play they can open up and create new ideas. Improvising is catching the moment, thinking and doing the unexpected (and sometimes paradoxical) and this is often what the couples need to get out of locked relationships and other relational problems.

Closely related to improvisation is play. Play as an "as if" activity – it is real for the player but not real, just fantasy or play for the outside observer. Play is also spontaneous and Wilson means this is a necessary part of creative improvisation.

Steve Harvey is a play therapist working with families and his model Dynamic Play Therapy, is a combination of *attachment theory* and *expressive arts therapy* (play therapy and dance therapy). Creativity for him is:

- Everyone has the ability to be creative
- Creativity is a combination of cognitive, motivational and affective elements related to each other
- The creative ability can be seen in the behaviour of the person and influences internal social experiences
- Creative abilities can be stimulated, be nourished and changed through *expressive arts therapy*
- In this therapy model movements, dramatic play, art and video are integrated (Harvey, 1990; 1994).

Jim Wilson and Steve Harvey work with children and their parents. It is very natural and obvious to use non-verbal observations and supporting parents to communicate with their small children in a developing and supportive way. It is equally natural and obvious to do family sessions with small and older children playfully using different play materials, with stuffed animals and dolls, and using fairy tales and metaphors. When talking about teenagers you have to abandon some of these "childish" behaviours and collaborate with them differently in a way that supports their shift to a juvenile identity.

When I first started to see couples, after many years of family therapy with children and their families and with adult addicts and their families, I was confused and couldn't really find out how to best carry out the sessions. I was not used to how aggressive, contemptuous and disrespectful some of the partners could be to each other. Family members more than often showed the care and the will to be of some help to each other.

It is fairly easy to get stuck, often in a similar way the partners are stuck, and of being drained of ideas and flooded by hopelessness. The chances to collaborate creatively diminishes and the session halts, stops or runs into the sand. If the therapist has a structure for the session (a map), but is not being too rigid about it, and at the same time allow her-/himself to be open minded, humorous, playful and thinking outside the box, the chances are good that the therapist and couple can meet and collaborate creatively. This must be done respectfully and can be described as serious play/improvisation and playful/improvisational seriousness.

Humour, playful thinking-and-doing, creative ideas, improvisations and unexpected questions and suggestions are very important parts of getting out of a problem and bringing forth new ideas. Timing is essential and crucial. Timing is all. The therapist's question or suggestion can be a disaster in the session if the timing is wrong, but the same question or suggestion can be constructive and helpful to the couple when the timing is right. If the couple and therapist/counsellor are attuned, then the window of collaboration and change is open.

Chapter 10

Coincidence Favours the Prepared Mind

Martin Söderquist

Reasons, Hopes and Goals

The couple counselling team in Malmö, Sweden is a small team of eight counsellors and the four authors of this book is the One at a Time (OAAT) team.

The service any team offer their clients must be organised in ways that fit the clients, the team and the organisation. In Malmö we have found that the following service offer suitable:

We offer couples several choices when they make appointments over the phone:

- Traditional couple counselling – the possibility to have several sessions with the same counsellor. This option involves a waiting list of several weeks and in periods of two to three months. It is the choice of 70–75% of couples. Two of the team members are specialised on sexual matters.
- OAAT – a session within a week. This is the choice of 25–30% of couples. There is the possibility to return for one or more sessions if the couple wishes it. If the couple schedule a new OAAT session, they are not guaranteed to see the same counsellor. Sessions are held on Tuesdays. Couples can schedule OAAT and also be put on the waiting list for traditional counselling. It is possible to cancel the traditional counselling if not needed after the OAAT session.
- One day multi-couple training day focused on conflict and communication
- One day multi-couple training day focused on sex and desire

We consider it important for couples to be given a choice. They know best what they need and want.

This goes for us counsellors too. The four of us are trained in family therapy, solution focused brief therapy and we have embraced the Single Session Therapy mindset the past ten years. But – we also have special interests and trainings - like Martin in Strategic Family Therapy and Family Play Therapy, Malena in Emotionally Focused Therapy and Lars and Karin in Gottman's method couple therapy. Counsellors do their best when being free to do what

DOI: 10.4324/9781003305774-10

fit them and the couples they see. We all have found that the solution-focused model is highly suitable when doing OAAT sessions, and we integrate our OAAT mindset with our special trainings and interests.

Our guiding principles in OAAT are:

- Having a choice
- Couples have different reasons for scheduling a session
- Couples know best how to move forward after the session
- Couples have hopes and goals for the OAAT session
- Context marking is of utmost importance
- Start from scratch knowing nothing about the couple in advance
- Being able to be genuinely surprised and giving hope

Couples choose OAAT for several different reasons. More than 1,200 couples (per year) schedule a session at Couple Counselling Team in Malmö, and

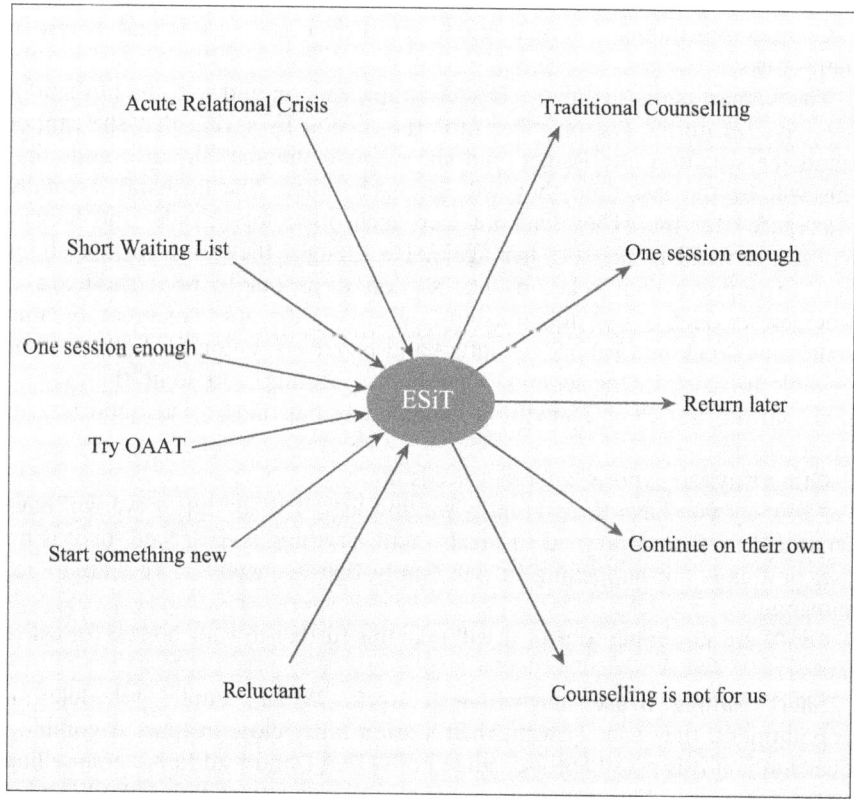

Figure 10.1 Summary of different options in OAAT including the possibilities for continued counselling

80% attend. As mentioned earlier, 27% schedule OAAT (Internal statistics, Couple Counselling Team, Malmö) and the majority attend one session. A total of 15% of those scheduling traditional counselling also attend only one session.

Why clients, couples and families schedule appointments at outpatient teams, emergency clinics and private practitioners are not always a wish for therapy and the reasons can vary a lot. Some years ago we interviewed the couples we saw about their reasons for choosing OAAT. These represent a great variety of reasons for their choice of OAAT.

Changes necessary now. In relational emergency or at a standstill in the relationship and with a necessity to get out of that situation and move forward, you do not want to hear when scheduling a session: "We have a three-four-month waiting list" or "You can have an assessment session".

According to de Shazer optimal time from scheduling the session to seeing the therapist is four to seven days (de Shazer, personal communication, 1994). This is what is expected by the client, but it is not always possible to offer this in different organisations.

Couples scheduling counselling express their urgent needs and hopes in many ways:

The woman had scheduled a OAAT couple session and told the husband a few days before the session. She starts the session by saying that she cannot stand the situation any longer, and she wants a divorce. She also adds that this will be the last time they will see each other. The husband is totally unprepared for this. They had not seen each other for a while, and he was looking forward to meeting her again. He thought they were to talk about how to improve their relation. The session turns out to be a sudden and emergent ending of the relationship – what for her was emergent became acute and shocking for him. A mutual and positive solution for both was not possible to reach in the session. They had a meeting, and some things were said that did not change anything immediately but maybe was important in the long run.

Other ways to express emergent needs are:

"You say you have three months waiting list? It is too late – we will have separated by then or argued so much that everything is destroyed, or it is no use, or things are happening in our family that are awful – we have to see someone."

Or: "I am not going to wait, I will take this further to your bosses! (or call a lawyer).

Short waiting list/session within a week. When couples schedule an appointment, they usually want their session fairly close in time. A common question is if it is possible to schedule both OAAT and traditional counselling at the same time. Our answer is of course. You can start with OAAT, and if you need continue with Traditional counselling or if you do not need it just cancel the appointment to Traditional counselling. Meeting the couples in this way is important as a positive service to them and we are very much aware of the fact that the OAAT session can turn out to be crucial. The scheduled Traditional counselling can be an assurance, although it might not be used. If the couple needs additional sessions a platform for continued positive collaboration will have already been created.

One of our clients said: "What calmed me down was that we could schedule and have an appointment so quickly" (Söderquist et al., 2018, in Swedish). Another couple told their counsellor: "Tell your bosses this was very good, and it is fantastic to have a session when you need it."

One session is enough. In a follow up study in Helsingborg, when I worked there (see Appendix), several couples said "one session was enough" and told us they got what they wanted or needed. Neither couples nor counsellors usually knew this in advance. If the couple needs additional sessions, they can of course return – it is up to them to schedule or not.

Following is an example from one of my sessions:

The couple began the session by asking if they could schedule several sessions. I told them this could be arranged – they could have another OAAT or schedule Traditional counselling. I also said: "Let us come back to this when we are to terminate the session today". In the session we talked about the family crisis they were facing last weeks. It was apparent to me early in the session that the couple had made a fantastic effort and told them: "You have done everything right, created something good for the whole family and done what could be expected from outside the family. You have achieved this in spite of all the work and the consequences for you as a couple" The couple said they were relieved and thanked me: "This was exactly what we needed and were hoping to hear". We continued the session discussing what they were planning to do ahead and how they could do this in practice. Last comment from the couple before they left the session room was: "We don´t need any more sessions. We were affirmed in what we both had been thinking and doing the right things."

Try counselling. It is not obvious therapy or counselling is the best choice for the couple. You can´t ignore the fact that all kinds of counselling and therapeutic sessions can be iatrogenic (Olsson and Petitt, 1999, in Swedish) even when the intentions are the best. When talking about Intimate Partner Abuse it is not recommended to have conjoint sessions if the violence is very dangerous and/or the perpetrator doesn´t take the responsibility for violating the integrity of his or her spouse.

Before a first session with a counsellor, clients and couples can be very insecure and even afraid. The chance of having one session as a try-out without committing to several sessions or long-term therapy should be a right for everyone.

Here follows one example how this can be expressed by a couple:

COUPLE: We don´t know if we are in the right place, but several of our friends have told us we should go to you. We were thinking of having a session to try if this fits us.

COUNSELLOR: Of course you can. Let us do the best of the session today and we will see if this is right for you. It might even turn out you don't need any more sessions. What do your friends see or hear that make them suggest counselling?

Start of something new. There are always ups and downs in all relations and sometimes everything goes round in circles. "We are not able to get out of this and it takes a lot of energy and power from us. We are not good enough for our children and each other – all of what we do is about handling everyday life". When love, will power and energy is there to try together finding a way back and proceed forward, OAAT can be a tool to break the grey or destructive pattern. Maybe the couple just need a little push in the right direction.

This quotation is from a session:

COUNSELLOR: What are your best hopes for the session today?
WOMAN: We are so bored, everything is routines and musts. We are stuck in vicious circles.
MAN: We need to get started with something that is good for us.
COUNSELLOR: Lets imagine you get hold of this tomorrow. What are the first thoughts and what do you start doing directly that tell you "we are getting out of the vicious circle and start finding what is good for us?"

Sometimes it takes a little bit longer in the session to get to the point where you can focus the small changes the couple are doing already to get out of the vicious circle and instead creating good circles.

Reluctant couples. Some couples are more reluctant. One of the partners might be experiencing their situation as awful and wants help, while his or her partner in no way can think of seeing a "shrink". Sometimes the help-seeking partner succeed in persuading the reluctant partner to **one** session but not several. The counsellor can express this in many different ways, when putting his or her first question to the couple. The question can be, for example "What can we do here today to make your situation/relationship better?" or "What are your best hopes for the session today?". The answers to these questions can be like this heterosexual couple told the counsellor in their OAAT session:

MAN: I don't know – I found a note on the kitchen table saying I was supposed to be here today at nine o'clock.
COUNSELLOR: You have had some time to think about this and here we are now. What are your thoughts?
MAN: I do it for her. I don't want to lose her.
    It can be like this too:
WOMAN: My husband really doesn't want to be here but I think we have to start talking.

The counsellor has several options for example ask the woman how she succeeded in bringing her husband to the session or ask her what she regards as necessary to start talking about.

Another example:

One of the partners starts the session by saying "I won't say a word in this session". The counsellor – surprised and astonished – laughingly says "This is rather uncommon in couple counselling. Are you OK with me talking to your partner and you just listening? If there is anything you want to disagree with or add – can you give me a sign?". Later in the session the counsellor asked the silent partner and got a fairly detailed answer.

There are many reasons why couples want to attend counselling sessions. In OAAT all reasons are acceptable. The couple can make a try and use the session in a way that is beneficial to them. It is important the couple experience they have a choice, they decide what happens in their lives and in what format they prefer their counselling.

It is equally important that couples after the session have several options like returning to OAAT, scheduling Traditional counselling, continue on their own, see the OAAT session as enough or decide: "counselling is not for us/ doesn't fit us". Sometimes a couple asks: "What do you think we should do? and they expect an answer. If the counsellor does not have an answer the best thing to do is telling the couple they have to figure out themselves. The counsellor cannot and should not decide what the couples are to do, but the counsellor can express an idea or give the couple a suggestion they can consider and later decide what to do.

Later in this book I will return to the question of counsellors' activity in giving suggestions and how these suggestions can be expressed.

There are many ways for couples to enter OAAT and there are many ways to move forward. This kind of flexibility is a very important part of OAAT.

Hopes and Goals

It can always be discussed what causes problems and what brings change. In OAAT with its awareness of restricted time we have found that it is most effective to focus what the couples hope for and what they want to achieve. The reasons they express (see above) are important – it sets the stage for the session - but even more important are their hopes and goals for the session, embedded in the problem descriptions. Example of this: The couple express their difficulties communicating, and the therapist asks both partners "What way of communicating would be better for you?" Focusing their ideas and hopes for something that maybe is achievable. I see this as the content and meaning of the session. The couples often want something but don't dare to mention and do not even expect it maybe. It is up to the counsellor to invite them to describe this. The couples hopes are expressed in so many ways, a broad palette of hopes and goals, and are idiosyncratic for them. It could be too great a challenge to go through them all.

To summarise: we try to keep the couple's reasons, goals and hopes in the foreground of our minds and focus descriptions of the couples doing. Problems, thinking and feelings expressed by the couples are of course important, but we try to keep this in the background. Focus on problems and feelings has a tendency to prolong counselling. Focusing descriptions of doing make it easier to find goals, exceptions and already made progress (de Shazer, 1982; 1988; 1991; de Shazer et al., 2007; Berg and Dolan, 2001) and explore and notice the competencies and resources of the couple and their strengths to resist oppression, violence and problem (Wade, 1997).

Context Marking and Starting from Scratch

Context marking is always important in every therapy or counselling. It is necessary for clients/couples and counsellor to negotiate and agree on who they are, what they are to do in the session and why the couple wish a session. The OOAT session might be the only one, and this makes it even more important to clarify all these questions. It is crucial to do this to make expectancies and hopes realistic and clarify what can be done in one hour. The context marking is at the same time an invitation to the couple to talk about what they want and hope for.

In our team we start from scratch – we never know anything about the couple apart from names, ages and any children they might have. We consider it important to hear the couple tell their story, what they want and what they hope for. Information from other persons before seeing the couple can be interesting but also misinform and lead the counsellor in directions not beneficial to the couple. This is why we want to see the couple without any beforehand information.

Genuinely Surprised and Giving Hope

We see couples with varied problems, different reasons for making an appointment and with unique hopes and goals - to paraphrase Forest Gump "*couple counselling* is like a box of chocolates – you never know what you get". To be prepared for everything, do the best of the OAAT session in collaboration with the couple and being able to be genuinely and positively surprised is extremely important for counsellors. Coincidence favours the prepared mind.

All affirmations and reflections made must be genuine and true. When made from a stance of positive surprise they are even more genuine.

The goal of the OAAT session is to bring the couple something new, like a new perspective on a problem and trying something different in a certain situation, The collaboration, the new stories, the possibilities can be created in the session. In the session the couple might find themselves describing things they have already done to solve their problems (and forgotten) and move forward, hear their partner tell things they never heard before and finding out what they want and need to do tomorrow. All this can give the couple hope for the nearest future and give them ideas of what they can do together. Hope might be the most important goal of therapeutic and counselling sessions.

Invitations and responses

We are all social beings and exist in relations. This means we are defined as persons and we develop in relations. No one is an island – we are all the time connected with others and in relationships. We interact and communicate in many different ways; non-verbally, by for example; gestures and eye and body movements, verbally by words expressed in all kinds of emotional states. When people meet, they cannot help interacting, it is natural and inevitable.

The process in these interactions can be described as initiatives and responses and as taking turns (Aarts, 1995). The child does or says something directly to or in the direction of the parent and the parent responds or not. Several initiatives and responses in a row are called Taking Turns, and this builds up the relationship.

I prefer to use the words Invitations and Responses. Invitations can be everything; a gesture, a word, a question, a problem description and a look in the eyes of the other. Responses are of the other looking back, answering the question, commenting on the words or not listening. The response is simultaneously an invitation to go on discussing, or to leave the subject or introducing something new. As "You never know what your question was until you get the other person's response" it is very important to be observant and sensitive to be able to continue to be on speaking terms and on the same interactional level with the other.

In the context of couple therapy the couple and the therapist make invitations: "welcome to our world" and "welcome to therapy or counselling" and they respond to each other in different ways. The couples present their problems, hopes and wishes which can be seen as invitations to the therapist to respond to and to do something about. The therapist invites the couple to discussions, reflections and problem solving or work things through depending on the preferred therapeutic model of the therapist. In the beginning of the sessions the couples and the therapists are negotiating what they are to do together in the session. The start of the session is very crucial – to avoid misunderstandings and collaboratively find a realistic common project.

There are a lot of challenges for the therapist when the couples invite the therapist into their world: Couples can present and invite the therapist to many different themes or problems, often seemingly contradictory, or embedded or directly expressed hopes and goals, and sometimes nothing at all with only one of the partners presenting something.

Different themes/problems. Not all problems can be solved in one session, and the response from the therapist needs to address this and focus on what can be collaborated upon in the session that can be useful and beneficial to the couple. This can be done with questions like. What is most important for you today? What do you think is the smartest thing to do – choose the problem to discuss in the session today that it is most likely to be able to do something about, or maybe choosing the most urgent problem? The therapist invites the couple to decide and at the same time invites the partners to focus on important, small and immediate goals.

Contradictory goals. Not all couples are in agreement, and they enter the session with different – and in many cases – contradictory hopes and goals. Not everything can be done in one hour. If the couple's goals are contradictory, it might be impossible to solve that problem. The therapist's response and invitation can be: Is it possible for you to come to an agreement on what to focus on in the session **today**? If we split the session in two and you get half an hour each to present your goals – how does that sound? If something happens today and you leave the session with a feeling of relief and joy – what would it be like for you?

One of the partners presents something, while the other is silent: Couple therapy is about the relationship and both partners need to be active in some way. The therapist has to ask questions to know if the partners agree on what their problems and goals are or if they have different goals. The therapist can ask the silent partner if it is OK to talk to the vocal partner and tells the silent partner: "If you don´t agree, or want to say something you are free to comment, is that OK?" The therapist can talk to the partner in terms of what would be different for her/him if the goals presented were reached and how that would be beneficial to her/his silent partner.

"This was not our idea": Some couples schedule an OAAT session after being persuaded by relatives, their teenage daughter, friends or in some cases being forced into it by the authorities. To know what to do in this session all three persons involved need to figure out who wants to see what changes and why. One way is to ask: "Suppose the session today is like a miracle and the person (s) that persuaded you to come here notices this. What will they notice?" Why do you think … . wanted you to schedule this session? Which person of all the people you know is the most eager to help you?

There are thousands of responses and invitations that are possible in every situation and my experience from couple therapy and counselling is that very often the first thing the couple say or do in the session is very important. The very first utterance is crucial and contains problem descriptions and embedded hopes and goals.

Some examples:

One of the partners begins the session (even before the therapist has welcomed them) by saying "I have lost my feelings for my partner". This is probably the reason why they have scheduled the session but most important is what the hopes and goals of the couple are. Do they want to come back to each other, or do they want to finish their relationship? Questions like: When did that happen? Do you think you can find your feelings again? When did you notice your partner lost her feelings for you? Do you think she will come back to you? The therapist follows the couple's lead and invites the partners to describe in more detail and simultaneously focuses what can be done in the one-hour session by questions like: If this session changes anything – what changes do you prefer? or "You can't force yourself but after this session you know what to do – what is different then?"

"We can't communicate or we fight all the time." This is of course not completely true. Apparently they decided together to schedule the session and they probably do not fight 24/7. The therapist can focus on situations and moments of agreement and positive communication by asking when and how they manage to create these moments. Is it possible to have more of these situations? Is that their embedded hope?

"Give us new ideas!" The couple present themselves as totally bereft of ideas and plead for help. The therapist needs to know how they have tried to solve their problems. It is not a good idea to give the couple ideas they have tried and failed (partly so at least). You can suggest several experiments and the couple can choose what fits them or you can present something that is unusual or surprising. Combined with humour and laughter these suggestions of doing something different can be both fun and changing. Toss a coin or dice next time you feel you are getting close to a quarrel or a fight is one example of a new idea. A variation of giving us new ideas is "You are the expert – we expect you to help us with this problem and solve it". This is most often unrealistic but necessary to be taken seriously. "I see myself as an expert of conversation and I will do my best this session and I suppose you will do the same to find out what can be your solution" is a reasonable response and invitation.

A final example: When invited by the therapist asking what their best hopes of the session today are, the couple becomes silent and after a while they or one of the partners say "I/we don't know". Don't know is very often implying the person needs more time to think and giving them time is probably the best response/invitation. Just wait and don't push – the session is a whole hour or one hour and a half. To everything there is a time.

There are lot of things to think of and take a stance. The most important aspects can be summarised:

- To enter the session and focus on this session and nothing else isn't taught in training for different therapeutic models more focused on processes and phases in therapy. The idea of a second session doesn't exist in OAAT and if/when the client/couple return for another session this session is a new one with new prerequisites. In solution focused brief therapy the session can be the last but in OAAT ideas of how to conduct this second and following sessions are outlined.

- To genuinely listen to the client/couple/family, what they want, what their goals are demand us to put our own ideas and agenda aside and really use the fact we have two ears and one mouth.
- To be flexible and open to the unexpected, negative and positive, is an advantage in OAAT. If the couples are locked up in relations that don't work for them it is good if the therapists aren't locked up in her/his therapeutic model. "Coincidence favours the prepared mind".
- To be open to many and different therapeutic models and having several different tools in your toolbox is an advantage for both clients and therapists.
- To restrain from doing too much and from having higher goals than the clients is not easy but necessary.
- To find balance between information overload and "what is realistic to reach today" can be a delicate task. You can't go for everything and all that is said in the session mustn't be analysed and deepened. The focus has to be on what is most important to the couples and what is reachable in the session.
- The biggest challenge of all; therapist and counsellors need to realise we are not so important as we sometimes think. Clients, couples and families are more successful than they know, and they manage a lot in everyday life. We can and should add something minor to them, but it requires quality and constructiveness to be helpful and achievable to them. The aim of the session is to help the clients having ideas of their way forward and in best cases having a plan to reach their goals.

It is impossible to do everything in one session. OAAT requires focus and concentration from both parts and what is important can't wait until next time because the OAAT session is the only one. Information overload needs to be put aside, all descriptions of clients' history and background aren't needed (no need for an archaeological dig) and the therapist have to lead and follow to make the session effective by staying in the present.

How to do this in practice and how to structure an OAAT session will follow in next chapter.

Chapter 11

Doing OAAT Counselling with Couples

Martin Söderquist

All therapies and series of sessions have a structure like: Before session, beginning of session, middle phase, ending and clients own continued work. See, for example, Hoyt, 2017.

Structure in General and in Detail

Before session. There is usually a longer period before a client reaches out for a therapist and sometimes emergent events make them schedule an appointment. Regardless of the time before session many things can happen in the life of the client. The client/couple thinks their situation/problems through, summarises and prepares for therapy. This often influences their lives positively. When they attend their first session they might already have begun thinking differently and doing things in everyday life that maybe is the start of solving their experienced problems. The couple has begun talking more than before and in a calmer and thoughtful way. Progress and changes are made before the first and often only session. This is necessary to notice and talk about in the session.

When clients enter the session room for the first time, they are not a clean slate. The therapy or counselling session is only a small part of their lives.

Beginning. The session continues in the same way as it begins. First contact is established and how to talk in the session and what goals the couple wish to be negotiated. Clients and therapists enter the therapy/counselling with different assumptions. The clients can be filled with hopes and expectations, looking forward to the start of processing their thinking and doing, they can be doubtful, nervous, worried or in direct opposition to all involvement in their family from outsiders. Depending on what the context and tasks of the therapist they might have been asked to assess the client, begin a series of therapy sessions, motivate the client to therapy, do a emergency session or manage a consultation interview. There are many variations of different sessions. One or few sessions are often regarded as a failure or drop out by many therapists, but this is not necessarily the case. The first and often only session is maybe enough for the client, or they think or tell in the follow-up session:

DOI: 10.4324/9781003305774-11

"Life came in between". There are lot of things to handle in everyday life for people, priorities to be made or positive events making therapy redundant.

Middle phase. The session continues from what has been said in the beginning and how the client has expressed and detailed her/his hopes and goals. The focus in the middle phase is on detailing and making the descriptions of the client's goals, plans and strategies concrete. The middle phase is therefore different and unique in every session.

Ending. It is optimal to end in a planned way and to together summarise; repeat client's strategies in case of relapse, plans for continued work and maintenance of progress and reaching goals and say goodbye. The ending is as important as the beginning - it ends an important phase in the life of the client (Hoyt and Rosenbaum, 2018). A clear and definite beginning and ending marks, makes it explicit and give the clients conditions to begin something new. The circle is closed.

In reality, endings are not so optimal as this. The client or the couple don´t show up for next session, cancel the session or don´t call. The clients continue their lives which is topic for next section.

Continued work by the clients/couples. The progress made in therapy stays with the clients or even continues over time. What the clients learned in therapy they can use in their everyday life. Of course, this is not always the case. Old habits die hard and some clients relapse but maybe not to where they were long ago, some clients enter therapy or get help in other ways to handle their new situation.

It is interesting how this overall structure for therapy is the same for a single session. There is a parallel between macro- and microcosmos. The same structure can be seen in One at a Time (OAAT).

Structure in Detail

Every counselling session is unique and is created collaboratively. No session is like other sessions. From this follows there is no manual or program for OAAT. To manualise would be abusing the ideas of Brief Therapy, Single Session Therapy (SST), Walk-in and OAAT. How SST sessions can be organised and structured is described in several publications (Hoyt et al., 2014; 2018; 2021; Paul and van Ommeren, 2013). OAAT team in Malmö is inspired of all these and we have accommodated these ideas to our OAAT practice with couples.

An OAAT session is as earlier mentioned a whole with a definitive beginning and ending. Ideas of continued sessions or next session should not exist in the mind of the therapist. All focus must be on the here and now. Because of this it is important beginning and ending are marked clearly and being ritualised.

If we divide the phases in a session in *beginning, middle and ending* it might look like this (of course, not all OAAT couple sessions include everything mentioned here):

Beginning – Find a Mutual Platform/Common project

- Context marking
- Most important today
- Hopes
- Goals
- Strengths and resources

Middle – Deepening/Widening Descriptions

- Pre session changes
- Exceptions
- Detailed descriptions of problems, tried solutions, small goals, and small steps in this direction
- Plans for the nearest future

Ending – Clarifying and Planning

- Summarising the session
- Ideas to bring home

When it comes to teamwork, this can be organised in many ways. For example, the team can observe the session from another room through mirror or on TV screen but they can also be in the session room. Some couples and clients prefer the team being in the room, they want to see and hear the team face to face. The situation is more personal they say. The task of the team varies in different therapeutic models (Hoyt et al., 2018; de Shazer et al., 2007; Andersen, 1991; Selvini Palazzoli et al, 1982; Söderquist, 2002, 2009b, in Swedish).

In our team sessions (not every Tuesday) we do not use pre-session discussion as many other single session teams do, as we do not know anything about the couples in advance. What we do is: the counsellor who is to conduct the session tells the team what help she/he wants and what comments on her/his way of conducting session she/he expects.

The tasks of the team (sitting in another room and watching session) are to carefully watch, notice and contribute with affirmations and ideas to the couple. These affirmations and ideas are discussed in the team discussion before ending the session. The counsellor talking to the couple summarises these discussions with the couple in the end of session. After session, when the couple have left, the team discuss briefly and we use a model we call *Two green and one yellow* when we give feedback – the conducting counsellor receives two affirmations (green) for constructive and helpful behaviour in the session and one (yellow) alternative idea/intervention from each team member.

Beginning. All kinds of sessions begin with welcoming. The couples are usually nervous, uncertain or irritated and need a friendly welcoming to make a landing in the session room and a good start. This often happens immediately in the doorway when couple and therapist say hello. Next step is to context mark (Petitt and Olson, 1992, in Swedish): clearly inform the couple of confidentiality, the structure of the session and negotiate who we are, what and why we are talking.

I usually do context marking like this:

"You are very welcome. My name is Martin. Do you have any questions to me, about couple counselling or OAAT before we proceed? (sometimes the couple do have questions; sometimes not). We guarantee absolute confidentiality; all we talk about in session stay in the room. We have to report to Child Protection if we get knowledge of children being in danger – for others like teachers, social workers, therapists it is enough with having suspicions of children in danger to report to Child Protection. I take notes to remember important details in our conversation, I want everything to be accurate. After session you can bring my notes home – they are yours, otherwise the notes are shredded. The session is approximately one hour - one hour ten minutes totally. After 45–50 minutes I will leave the room to go through the session myself. This will give you some minutes to reflect, talk to each other or just take a break. I will be back after seven minutes or so to summarise my reflections on your situation and if I have what I see as good ideas to suggest to you I will present these ideas. It is you who decide if these ideas are fit for you. OK?"

"I know your names....you are.... old and have ... children. I never know more than this in advance – I want to hear from you. We have agreed on one session – let us do our best together to make it as useful as possible to you!"

This is how I begin sessions and do context marking and my colleagues do their idiosyncratic variations of this. In other contexts, it will be different of course.

The continuation of session can vary a lot but in all sessions the client and therapist need to agree on the aims and goals of the session. It is important to use the session effectively to enhance the chances for couples to get affirmations and the help they need. Alternatives for continued session can be structured by following questions (they can also be used in individual and family sessions).

- How come we are sitting here today? Please tell me why you are here?
- What are your best hopes for the session today? What are you hoping to get from the session?
- Imagine one hour from now. You are leaving the session room and are very satisfied with what we talked about/ what you received – what is different? How do you notice?
- There are two themes I want to focus on in the session; the problem that has brought you here and most of all what you hope for from this session? Which do you prefer to begin with?

The importance of humour cannot be overestimated. Regardless of whatever techniques the therapist/counsellor have in their toolbox acceptance, treatment and respect are most important and crucial to help the couple gain confidence and trust. Combined with humour – the ability to laugh together, relax and free creativity it will help the couple to view situations in other perspectives. It is possible to affirm the seriousness of the couple's problems and situations, listen and try to understand and simultaneously use unexpected questions, see things from another angle and notice and affirm the good and normal things the couple think and do. Telling the couple about other couples (of course with their permission), of experienced situations in other sessions or using metaphors can be normalising and give new or surprising perspectives. When couples say: "We have not thought like this before" or laughingly tell you "Are we strange or mad when we do like this?" they acknowledge they can see openings and possibilities ahead. "Nothing is so serious you can´t laugh at it", comedians used to say, and when being done in sessions respectfully and in collaboration, the sessions are easier and more constructive to the clients. Several therapists have written about humour in therapy (Cade and O´Hanlon, 1993; Cade, 2014; Baruch Shulem, 1988, Hoyt and Andreas, 2015; Andreas and Hoyt, 2016). Humour is maybe the royal road to problem solving in economy and politics. Amos Oz's (2010) view of the matter is that humour in combination with the ability and willingness to look at the existence with the eyes of the other is what is necessary to solve problems and find compromises. The ability and willingness to look at things with the eyes of the other is not about understanding it is about trying to understand. Steve de Shazer used to say that we can´t understand each other but we can creatively misunderstand each other (de Shazer, 1991).

The importance of humour in therapy and the risk of humour being misunderstood is illustrated in this brief story from a training group:

"Many years ago I attended a training day with NLP (Neuro-linguistic programming) and the trainer presented a video. The client and the therapist laughed a lot in the session and some of the participants got irritated and were agitated. They said the therapist in the video session wasn´t serious and didn´t understand and affirm the client. I was thinking the laughing was a bit overwhelming, but I saw and heard the client being affirmed and having some new ideas. Serious problems must not always be met with wrinkled forehead, leaning head and hypnotic voice I said to myself a bit naughtily. Most important is to meet the clients where they are and help them proceed in their lives."

The couples enter therapy and bring to the sessions what they see as huge problems and the therapist need to listen carefully and affirm. Is not unusual the couple begin with: "We want to tell our story/our problems/our background for you to understand". This is of most importance to the couple, but time does not allow this to be the sole focus of the session. One way to meet this request is, before they begin their story, briefly ask them what they want you to listen for especially and what they want you to make of the information they give you.

Another common scenario is when the couple after a series of questions tell you "We don't really know". This answer is usually an expression for "We need more time". The therapist/counsellor doesn't have to press or hurry in this situation – there is time and space to ask questions, think and reflect: "We have a whole session", as Bobele and Slive (2014) put it: One example:

"The couple had problems describing what they hoped for in the session and after a while I asked them to think three months into the future when they see my colleague in traditional counselling and told them: You tell the counsellor the relational changes you have accomplished after the OAAT session. You even think you didn't need any more sessions or not so many. What do you tell my colleague counsellor?"

In an OAAT session, it is of utmost importance that the affirmations, clarity, listening and humour are combined constructively to make the session useful to the client/couple. Most often it is the only session they will have.

The content of the beginning presents a smaller amount of situating and perspective questions and with more focus in the beginning and middle phase of the session on the here and now and nearest future - possibilities and initiatives questions (see Chapter 6, Hornstrup, Tomm and Johansen model).

Same structure as in other formats of therapy/counselling but OAAT does not focus what has been instead the focus is now and the nearest future.

Middle phase: In this phase the couple and the counsellor build more and detailed descriptions of what the couple express as the most important to them in the session today and what their goals are. Collaboratively couple and counsellor define and deepen the couples descriptions of hopes, aims and goals. This part of the session is unique for every couple and session. The counsellor must closely follow the couple, listen and asking and be careful not to express his or her own ideas to quickly. The same goes for individual and family sessions.

The questions from the counsellor can be varied and the aim of them is to help the couple describe their situation, their problems, their hopes and their goals in detail:

- What have you been trying so far to solve your problems?
- What is different after you made the appointment?
- What is different last week?
- Who will be the first one to notice when something in your relationship develops in the right direction?
- What will be the first sign of success in talking constructively and not ending up in quarrels like you did before?
- What do you individually want more of in your relationship?
- What can you do together to make this happen?
- What are your plans to make your relationship better?
- What can/will your individual contribution be?

The questions can be varied endlessly and from above you can notice all of Karl Tomms questions are included – questions referring to history/past and future as well as co-clarifying and co-constructive questions. OAAT is future- and action-directed and focuses on possibilities and initiative questions.

Now is the time to mention the concept *exception*. In early solution-focused literature, exception was sometimes defined as instances or moments of problems not existing or dominating.

This definition is grounded in the problem, and I call these exceptions *problem-related. Goal related exceptions* on the other hand are instances and moments where parts of these moments are how the couple wants life to be like. The two kinds of exceptions can be correlated but mustn´t necessarily be so. The absence of something is not the same as presence. This can be confusing in couple sessions.

Examples of different question:

When asking the couple if they argue and fight all the time, they of course answer "No". They go on with describing how they get exhausted and tired and therefore stop fighting. However, if the counsellor's questions are competence- and future-oriented and focused on what the couple see themselves doing together when they are satisfied with their lives and their communication runs smoothly, they will describe very different behaviour and feelings.

To be free from problems is what the client wants, but her/his goal is sometimes something else. A couple constantly fighting do not do this all the time (problem-related exceptions) but explain this away, do not notice or say that it does not count. What they want and hope for – their goals – are to appreciate, see and love each other (goal-related exceptions). In sessions where you focus on problem-related exceptions – the absence of problems – it takes longer to reach descriptions of goals. There is the risk of looking where you do not find what you are looking for, and the session will not be useful to the client.

In sessions focusing goal related exceptions, presence of the already acquired, done in the here and now or possible to do more of in the future – the chance for easier access to clients' descriptions of goals will be greater and together we find a way to make the session useful. Goal related questions, best hopes at the moment, wishes for tomorrow and scaling questions 1–10 are focusing the future (what the client can and is willing to do) and the clients preferred direction to reach her/his goal. These kinds of questions possibly lead the conversation to exceptions, resources and what the couple can do as the first step to reach their goals.

It is also important to couples that the session is about the right themes and leads to what they want and therefore the counsellor needs to ask them; "Are we on the right track?", "Are we talking about the things you want and need?", "Are my questions helpful?" or "I have several ideas how we can continue the session. Please allow me to present them to you and then you can decide".

In the middle phase, it can be helpful to couples when the counsellor introduces what is known from research on couples' relationships. In our team we have been inspired by Gottman's research and evaluations (Schwartz-Gottman and Gottman, 2015). Depending on what the couple present as their problems and goals the counsellor tell them relevant facts from research.

Examples:

Sound relationship house. Couples need a stable relational platform to be able to solve their conflicts and to enhance their relation. Some couples need to start from the beginning – getting to know each other again, beginning to appreciate and affirm each other. Some couples already have this relational platform, and the session can more directly focus solving conflicts. When looking together at the house the couple can scale how much they have on each floor for example. They can also bring the picture of the house home as a reminder.

Emotional account. In every relationship it is necessary to put in more than you withdraw. Communication is always directional: towards, turning against and turning away. Turning towards is to look each other in the eyes, respond, be kind, comment appreciatively and this leads to understanding, mutuality and participation. Turning towards is input in the relation. Turning against is to criticise, go against, verbally abuse and accuse and turning away is not answering, to turn away and not care about and all this is withdrawal from the account. These withdrawals can be devastating to the couple, if the communication is unfriendly or aggressive and in a heightened emotional tone. The Gottmans say the input/withdrawal coefficient need to be at least 5:1, every withdrawal need five inputs if the couple will have a chance to handle problems of everyday life and be able to enhance their relationship (Schwartz-Gottman and Gottman, 2015). Useful questions: How do your inputs and withdrawals look like? How do see and appreciate each other? How do you show your love? How do you support each other and how do you express yourself when your partner does things you do not like?

A good start. It is not what you say it is how you begin communication/session that can be very crucial. By expressing in I-words and with a low and calm tone what you want instead of using the words you and never/always, the chances for a calmer and useful proceeding are enhanced. In the OAAT session the couple can role play different ways of starting conversations.

Importance of listening. This has been said before and important to focus on again. Giving time to let the partner talk and express what they want, not interruping and genuinely trying to understand your partner.

The couple seemed to be unable to listen to each other and they interrupted each other all the time. I couldn't hear what they said, and I got confused – what did they want from the session?

I came up with a suggestion to the couple: "I interview you individually for 15 minutes each and the one not being interviewed were to listen carefully without saying anything at all until they were to reflect.

They agreed, and we did the interviews. We all laughed together when one of them interrupted and I and the partner being interviewed simultaneously turned to her and gave her the yellow card (a warning in soccer; a foul in basketball).

Conflict curve. According to Gottman 70% of all relational conflicts can´t be solved and it is meaningless to try to do something about them (Schwartz-Gottman and Gottman, 2015). You had better focus on what is possible to handle and solve. You can draw the conflict curve on the whiteboard and collaboratively with the couple identify the most critical points (triggers, peak of conflict and getting connected again). This can be very useful to the couples to see. How they succeed and what they can do more of can give them ideas of how to do next time they end up in a conflict. For example, a couple might have good ideas of their triggers and how to avoid catastrophes but are not so good at reconnect after the fight. A variation is the window of tolerance. The focus in session can be the partners similarities and differences in handling their conflicts – fight, flight and freeze – when conflicts reach a level of too much (Siegel, 1999).

Repair Attempts (I sometimes call this The White flag). In all conflicts one or both partners try to stop or slow down but this is not noticed by the partner. It is maybe expressed in a lame or weak way or the partner is not receptive in the moment. Helping the couple find mutual white flags might be what they really need. A gesture, a word or a symbol might be good. One couple told me: "We can´t use the stop sign – we are police officers! We have to find something else".

There are many more therapists and researchers having described useful facts. We are also inspired by ideas other therapists have presented:

Good habits. It is very easy to create habits and patterns individually and in relations. Sometimes these habits and patterns turn into bane and bad habits. Introducing new and good habits take time and demand purposefulness. Stefan Klein describes this as constructing a new highway close to the old one. Until the new highway can be used properly your old habit easily forces you to slip back to the old highway (Klein, 2005, in Swedish). According to Lally et al. (2009), 66 days is the average time it takes to create a new habit and replace the old one. There are lots of examples of habits that can be changed by will and purpose. Individual habits like physical training, eating and idiosyncratic ways of behaving. Relational patterns like one partner always responding in a certain way when her/his partner expresses something which is followed by a discussion or a conflict much like a written manuscript. To replace deeply rooted patterns of behaviour like drug and alcohol addiction and criminal behaviour with newer and more constructive behaviour will of course take more than 66 days. OAAT can be the help the couple need to start in new directions but that doesn´t imply the counsellor have to join them for 66 days.

Transitions/Set time. A common human problem is everyday life including work, children, renovating houses and other additional stresses which can halt recovery. Everything just circles around over your head and transitions end up floating around and become unnoticed. The set time is missed. (Jönsson, 2005). The counsellor can help the couple stick to one item at a time when talking in the session as a way of introducing this.

Breaking patterns. Couples sometimes end up in patterns they cannot escape from and despite tremendous efforts they can´t succeed. Something new need to be introduced and this can be done in many ways. For example, Talk-Listen exercise can be tried in the session or the couples ideas of what could be done differently could be discussed. Introducing questions like: "What would your child (not the childs responsibility but children often come up with constructive ideas) say you two need to do in your situation?" or "Imagine ten years into the future and you remind yourself of what happened today – what are your best memories and how did you solve your problems?" can be very useful.

The couple were furious, very angry and argued loudly and I couldn´t stop them it seemed. After a while (at least twenty minutes!) I raised my hand and they looked at me with surprise and I asked if I could say a word. They agreed. I asked them the Miracle question (de Shazer, 2007) and suddenly the couple silenced and started reflecting.

Ending. Ending the session starts already in the beginning of the session when the counsellor asks the couple of their best hopes for the session. Ending is present all the time since the aim is to help the couple having a plan of action for their nearest future when leaving the session.

At the end of middle phase and in the end the focus is on the couples plans to go on their own and what both partners contribution to this will be. The questions are initiative questions in Tomm's words. At the end of the session, these plans and ideas are detailed and summarised. The end of session need to be clearly marked, and it is necessary that the couple leave the session with a feeling of "we really got something out of this". If they ask for tools or reflections from the counsellor, it is of utmost importance the counsellor respond. This can be done by putting the focus on the most important themes and exercises in the session combined with the counsellor giving the couple ideas to practice and continue implementing when home. Ending is to summarise and collaboratively point to the direction forward.

The following are different ways of asking questions to focus ending:

- It is getting time to summarise and end the session. Let us do this toge-ther. What has been most important to you and what do you take home from the session?
- Before we terminate the session – what will you take home and continue doing?
- Have we been talking about things you wanted and what was important to you?
- Before I leave the room to go reflecting on my own – this will give you some minutes to do your reflections – is there anything else you have

come up with? (it is common I myself come up with something I have forgotten when I ask this question).

- What will you most of all appreciate me telling you when I come back after my reflection time?

The summarising of the session must not be prolonged and no new session is to begin. The couple must of course have the chance to point out if anything has been missed or they have come to think of something during session. The counsellor has to respond to this and emphasise their continued work in everyday life. Often couples reflections and comments are very fascinating. Sometimes unexpected comments are made, sometimes - forgotten by counsellor and the partners - details in the session are mentioned and sometimes a request for continued sessions are made. As mentioned earlier it is always possible for the couples to schedule a new OAAT session, but they are not guaranteed to see the same counsellor next session.

The biggest difference between OAAT and traditional counselling is how the ending is handled. OAAT ends with the counsellor saying: "Good luck!" to the couple – a clear marking and not an indication of continued sessions. A brief sentence of two words expressing: We are finished, it was nice to see you, I wish you all the luck with what you think and plan ahead.

In more traditional sessions with continued sessions being planned or agreed it is more common with expressions like: "Time is out – lets continue next session", "See you next session", "Do you want to schedule a new appointment" or "Come back to me when you have given more thoughts to what we talked about/carried out your plans". These phrases/expressions are invitations to continued therapy.

Affirmations. Through the session the counsellor is continuously giving affirmations by cheering-up comments (a few, not too many), curious questions and reflections in the moment. This is what create the momentum and is the contribution by the counsellor to the "therapeutic dance".

A summary of the session is necessary to make a collaborative and constructive ending.

The couple need to get affirmations and confirmations to know that the counsellor has listened to what they have described of problems, goals and efforts. The counsellor can do this by having "individual reflection time by leaving the room for some minutes" or inviting the couple to collaboratively summarise the session. In the original literature (de Shazer, 1988) the summary is often described as being composed of compliments and tasks. I prefer to call what I do in the end of session *a summary of the session* as I see it and *reflecting back* to the couple my ideas I think could be useful to them. I seldom use the word compliments because this word implies a description of what the other person is for example looks, intelligence, characteristics and so on. Eastside Family Centre differentiate compliments and commendations (McElhcran and Harper-Jacques, 1994; Limacher and Wright, 2006). When I affirm that I want to point out to the couple what I have seen and heard the couple telling me, their different ways of handling their everyday life, their efforts to handle their problems and how they despite their crisis have been able to stay together. The affirmation is about the efforts of the couple and is a requirement for the counsellor to be able to present ideas as to what the couple can do.

The summary – affirmations and ideas – have different purposes:

- Mark the ending of session (brings the session to the end)
- Reflecting back to the couple (always wanted by couples)
- Leave the continued work to be done by the couple (pointing in direction of future)

In my book *Jag känner mig normal nu!* (Söderquist, 1995, pp. 159–162, in Swedish, with its title translated to English is *I feel normal now!*) a consultation with a mother and daughter, not uncommon in our practice as couple counsellor in Sweden, is described with a dramatic display of the importance of a summary being made:

"Antonia is 18 years old and just before session had been in emergency care following a suicidal attempt. No one sees her abuse of hashish or anorexia nervosa as being her real problem. All including her therapist share the belief that Antonias problems are related to her being sexual abused.

During the first 15 minutes of the session the mother and therapist put a lot of questions to Antonia and she makes some efforts to answer but the only answer she can produce is "I don´t know".

The situation in the room is more and more desperate. Mother cries out desperately "You must talk about it. You must talk about it Antonia", and Antonia shows that she is becoming more and more desperate: "Everyone is nagging me to talk about the abuse but I do not want to and I don't need it either" The atmosphere of desperation in the session room goes through the mirror to the observation room and the team and consultant don't know if they should postpone the session, refer to an emergency unit or try something quite different. They decide to try something different, there was nothing to lose, and the consultant (Martin Söderquist) enters the session room.

MS: When I see and hear you talk I came up with two ideas I want to share with you Antonia. The first is I came to think of glass doors – like entrances of shopping malls. If they are very well cleaned there is always a risk of bumping into them, you don´t see them. I think you have put such glass doors around you to mark who you are and to protect your integrity. I think this is good you do this. It is healthy.

Antonia looks up and looks MS in the eyes.

MS: Your mother and therapist who really are making efforts to help you unfortunately bump into the glass door since it is so well cleaned.

Mother nods in agreement, and Antonia keeps looking at MS and maybe nods.

MS CONTINUES: My second idea is – I would like to write a certificate of health because you have learned to protect your self and in a very clear and healthy way show your environment what you want and what you do not want and you know what you need.

Mother (reacts first: So good to hear you say this. So good. A stone fell from my breast (and she puts her hands on her chest. Antonia reacts by gazing with big eyes and with a teardrop slowly dripping from her eyes. Mother and daughter hug and cry together).

The therapist and the consultant leave the room to let mother and daughter have their moment on their own.

After some minutes they return and tell mother and Antonia:

MS: We decided to write a certificate of health. Here you are.

Antonia receives it and reads it through very carefully. The certificate says: *We hereby certify you are not half as sick as other people say.*

The session is ended, and later when scheduling the next session with the therapist, Antonia says: "This was the best thing ever. I will put the certificate in my folder for the important things in life. I will look at it when things are too rough."

When Antonia and her mother return for another session two weeks later Antonia is fine. She looked at the certificate in her folder twice these two weeks. She reports she has been able to preserve her integrity several times and she and her mother are in agreement: Antonia doesn't need a session next two months. Mother commenting: "Went straight into my heart".

During the session we were in danger of only seeing the hopelessness and difficulties and thereby diagnosing and seeing Antonia as sick. What Antonia most of all needed was to be told she wasn't so sick and that she deserved concern and to be noticed.

Pictures and metaphors can be very strong and affirming with perfect timing and fit and can help client and therapist to meet, understand and see each other. The reverse is also evident: if there is no fit the alliance will be negatively affected. The client will experience not being understood and the metaphor/picture can be very hard to erase.

In this case the intervention was given to a mother and daughter but an intervention similar and adjusted to the couple's situation – a couple with a traumatised partner and a very worried and scared partner – is of course possible in couples work.

Ideas and suggestions. Steve de Shazer once said he after careful investigation of many therapists interventions had come to the conclusion there are 165 different and possible therapeutic interventions (de Shazer, 1989, personal communication). This is a huge toolbox if you want to use it. Opinions are divided when talking about therapeutic interventions. Should interventions be used and if so how? Or should therapists refrain from interventions and letting the clients themselves come up with what to do? After training over the years with communication therapy, strategic family therapy and solution focused brief therapy I have found interventions, tasks and homework assignments a natural part of my therapeutic work with clients, couples and families. Structural family therapists stress the interventions to be made when there is high intensity in session and the aim of intervention is for the client to go on using at home what has been talked about in session (Minuchin, 1974). Strategic family therapists use the session to collect descriptions of behavioural sequences and interventions given are often paradoxical (Haley, 1973, 1976). In the world of systemic therapy quite early a difference appeared between Palazzoli recommending *invariant prescription* (Palazzoli et al., 1978) and Cecchin and Boscolo focusing *circular questions* as most important change tool (Cecchin, 1993).

The same discussion exists when coming to solution focused therapists – some therapists always suggest tasks and ideas to clients and some therapists don't even think about it, they regard the interview/conversation as being the most important (de Shazer et al., 2007).

There are those saying clients never follow the advice and tasks suggested by the therapists, and that is why it is useless to use interventions in this way. This is not true, I believe. Many couples benefit from ideas, exercises and information. Some couples listen to what the counsellor say and suggest, think it over and do their own variation. Some couples don´t do anything that the therapist says, but if presented as an idea or suggestion, they might give it a thought. If the suggestion does not fit the couple, they are the ones deciding what to do with it. This is no problem – an idea or suggestion is just an idea or suggestion, but if the idea is presented as homework this implies "must be done and reported".

Following is an example from a session where the therapist's suggestions wasn´t followed but however influenced the couple in a positive way:

I supervised two couple counsellor – live and being in the session room together with them and the couple. The man lost his temper easily and exploded after miniscule events and this affected his wife seriously and he hit the woman on occasions. The counsellors discussed with the couple these situations, their reactions and what they did. At the end of session the counsellors and I took a break to discuss what feedback we were to give the couple. We also had some ideas what to suggest to the couple what they could try at home together and especially what the man could try. Our idea that which we suggested was like this: Figure out six alternatives for behaviour/

what to do when getting furious and angry – one being what he usually did in these situations (this must still be an option), one alternative being secretive towards his wife and four alternatives which were to be discussed and decided collaboratively. Every morning he was to throw the dice and the number showing was to be his alternative behaviour that day, if he got furious and mad.

Next session the counsellors asked him, and he told them he hadn´t thrown the dice, but a day or two after last session he was stressed and in bad mood and thought: "If I trip on these bloody shoes always being in my way in the hallway, I will get mad, and this will not be a good thing for my wife". He decided to take an extra walk around the block before going home to calm down. This was one of the alternatives he and his wife had decided upon.

Homework assignments and tasks are not important and no ends in themselves, they are what the couples ask for and the counsellor having the idea. This means the idea has to fit the couple and must be custom-made to the couple's problems and goals.

The concepts task or homework assignment are often used and to many clients these words remind them of and evoke bad memories from their years in school. Structural and strategic therapy use the word *homework* (Minuchin, 1974; Haley, 1976) and Selvini Palazzoli and her colleagues use the word *intervention* (Boscolo and Bertrando, 1993; Selvini Palazzoli et al., 1981). Solution focused brief therapy use the word *task* (de Shazer, 1982; 1988; 1991; de Shazer et al., 2007).

I prefer the words *idea, suggestion or experiment* because they are more open, more generous and less forcing. I always tell the couple they are in the driver seat and it is their decision – if my idea fit (or not). The same goes for the concept break – the therapist leaving the room for individual reflections or discussions with team. I prefer the concept "*individual time for reflections*". I move (getting more creative), go through the session in my head and return to the couple with reflections and ideas. While I am out the couple is given the chance to do their own reflections. The concept break implies the counsellor doesn´t do anything or having a coffee and that is not the case. The individual time for reflection is often the most valuable part of the session.

Ideas and suggestions can be very varied:

Do more of what works. Already before session the couple are doing good things for themselves without knowing or noticing and the counsellor can suggest they observe when they behave like that or continue doing what they do since it seems to work fine. Counsellors suggestions can be for example – observe all small signs of moving forward in your relation/enhancing relation/all continued signs of what the partner does to improve their relation/all signs of efforts and attempts. Similar suggestions can be given clients or families of course.

Do something different. Sometimes couples are caught up in patterns and rigid behaviours and they can´t get out of it even when they know it is destructive to them. It can be helpful to them and give the counsellor ideas when talking in session what could be different behaviour. For example the counsellor can say something like: "Next time you get stuck in a situation I suggest you, both of you, do something different, something you know your partner would appreciate." I once suggested a father to do a rain dance instead of shouting and telling his son in a firm voice next time the son provoked him. Later the father told me he had done what I suggested and the previously unavoidable fight was replaced by a very surprised son and no fight. I told this story to a couple and they said: "We get your point but we have to find something else".

Breaking patterns. Sometimes couple end up in destructive patterns they can't break like "I must have the last word" or "I need to decide and not be controlled by you". A variation of "Odd days – even days" (Selvini Palazzoli et al., 1978) is when the counsellor suggests that the couple splits the week in two – odd days are one partners, even days the other partners. When it is their days, the partner in charge has the last word in discussions or can decide what to do when in an argument. In that way, both partners get 50% of last words or decision-making instead of constantly being discontent or feeling "never being right".

Don't fix what isn't broken. Sometimes the best thing to do is to not interfere, or as the Danes say "blande sig udenom" (mix and keep outside/stay out), and not ask questions or make suggestions. This is especially important when the clients very clearly are uninterested or do not see any problem at all. The counsellor can confirm their situation, affirm them for being persistent and fighting or something else the couple has mentioned in session but refrain from giving the couple any ideas. We know therapy is helpful to clients regardless of therapeutic model but there are always dangers involved in everything we do. Iatrogenic damages (Olsson and Pettit, 1999, in Swedish) can come into existence in therapy too. The experience of bad treatment, not being listened to and not being part of what really matters to you are examples of these kind of damages. This causes reduced or even diminished confidence in therapy or for the therapist for a lengthy period of time or perhaps forever.

Our team in Malmö has translated (with permission from Gottman) some of Gottman Institute material. We use Sound Relationship House, getting to know each other, talk – listen exercise, sex and desire cards as well as material from others as good habits and conflict curve in our sessions. These exercises and cards are suitable for couples to receive and use at home (Internal material, Couple counselling team in Malmö, 2010–20).

We have been inspired by others who have done evaluations and research on couple and in some cases translated and also produced own material we have found useful. How to create good habits (Lally et al., 2009), tolerance window (Siegel, 1999), talking with children when parents separate and meeting places/situations of connection and closeness in everyday life are examples of this (Internal material, Couple counselling team in Malmö, 2010–20).

There are more variations of what we use in sessions which the couples can take home: we use the whiteboard a lot in our team, we note the themes, goals and resources we talk about in session and nowadays the couple have mobile phones and it is easy to take a photo of the whiteboard. Sometimes I hand over my written notes on paper to the couple if they want it and if they can read what I have written (my handwriting is awful). Most important is that the couple take home what they want and need.

A brief story exemplifying this:

I was doing a consultation interview with Eva. She had been homeless for many years, and I took notes as usual. Eva was very affected by her hard life and experiences and had problem remembering things. She said her last days had been better: she stayed at a shelter, and she had met Jesus. We talked for a long time about this. After the session she told her contact person and the other persons at shelter she had experienced something fantastic – even better than Jesus. A week later she asked her contact person to help reading my notes – she had forgotten and wanted to refresh her memory of the session. She said she couldn't read my notes and her contact person told her: I can help you – I am in training with Martin, and I have learned to decipher his handwriting.

Nowadays there are many evaluations and research in different areas and on relations useful to couples regardless of where and who they see in sessions. It might be important to couples to look through this kind of material and take home. The Gottman cards are appreciated by the couples we see. The couples find them interesting, useful and the cards are reminders to them of what they need to focus in their relationships. This is different from client themselves trying to find material on internet which they might not be able to rely on.

The combination of questions, reflections, exercises, summaries, ideas/suggestions and material to bring home have the potential to make the sessions intensive, varied and give the clients what they want and need.

Creativity and Improvisation in Action with Couples

It is difficult perhaps even impossible to be creative or spontaneous on demand or on order. It is paradoxical – if you are spontaneous on demand, you are not spontaneous. It is the same with creativity. If someone comes up with creative ideas – where did it come from? Was it entirely from the person who expressed and presented the ideas or was it the discussion and social interaction that laid the ground for new ideas? The moments of creativity are collaboratively created in social interactions.

In couple therapy this collaboration can be difficult. Triangles are hard to manag,e and there are many challenges for the therapist and for the couple. The couple trying hard to force the therapist to take sides and becoming some sort of judge – deciding which of the partners is right in their dispute, is an example of this.

As mentioned in previous chapters, couples schedule OAAT for many reasons and present problems of all kinds. In Michael White's words they present *problem saturated narratives* (White, 1989). They describe being stuck in destructive patterns, angry feelings, contempt, hopelessness and many other problems and negative feelings. The strength of all this can be overwhelming for the therapists and the consequences can be destructive for a collaboration. This is of no help for the couples who need to be listened to but also want to see the light in the tunnel and get some new perspective. The therapist needs to listen carefully to the couple but stay out of the couples´ problems but not go too deeply into the problems to stay free. "Problem distance but not social distance". When the therapists are free, they can ask questions and reflect from an understanding, benevolent and friendly outside position focusing on the goals and hopes that are embedded in the problem descriptions. The couple start by saying "We want long term couple therapy". OAAT is not the right place for this but embedded in their request is "We want to change our relationship" and this is what the OAAT therapist can focus on.

Creativity thrives in gentle, open minded, positive atmospheres.

Couples often have ideas of what couple therapy is and what they think they can expect when in therapy. Sometimes couples feel therapy is the right kind of help at the right time, sometimes couples might have other expectations of what therapy can do and could feel frustrated. There is therefore a need to clarify the context of therapy at the beginning of the session.

The supposition of the crucial importance of talking about the problem and finding out the causes of the problem can be such a common misunderstanding. The couples have most probably talked a lot about this, discussed in detail, been fighting over it and talked to friends about it. They need something else and new to be able to see their situation differently and start constructive interactions.

Therapists introducing and inviting the couples to something unexpected and positive for the couples are puncturing the negative expectations and the problem focus. This can start a positive collaboration and open up space for creative possibilities and there are many ways to do that.

Dramatic and creative improvisation. Improvisation is spontaneous and doesn't follow rules or manuals. Every couple therapy session is unique and what is said and done in the session gives associations and ideas to those involved. Playback therapy (Wilson, 2018) is when the therapist reflects back to the family by taking on the roles of the family members and carrying out a role play. In a couple session (if you are two therapists) the two therapists can execute the role play with the couple as observers. Afterwards the couple can reflect and comment on the therapist's actions.

Sometimes the couple have trouble deciding what to do and how to make an important decision. Head (what they think they ought to do) and heart (what they feel is the right thing to do) are in a battle inside each partner and in the relationship. The therapist can suggest them to be the Head or the Heart and do a brief role play (Wilson, 2018).

Humour is freeing and a help to get rid of anxieties and tensions. Everything can be joked about, but it is important the couple and the therapist laugh together and not at someone's expense. When entering the session room one of the partners loudly says: "I don't want to be here". With a smile the therapist can answer: "With a weather like this outside – I agree. Let us do a Walk & Talk session" or "Me neither but now that we are here – let us do something together you can both benefit from". There are numerous examples of constructive humour in couple therapy sessions but caution and timing are recommended. It is not stand-up comedy or entertainment – couple therapy is a serious business.

One more example: Many years ago, long before I began working with SST/OAAT, I asked Ben Furman[1] to make a consultation with me, with the couple and the husbands´ family of origin. The couple and I had been going on and on with session after session and we couldn´t come to the point of terminating the therapy. Ben made the consultation in the same humoristic way as he always does, and when we were to terminate the session, he suggested the following: the couple were to stand up and the reflecting training group members were to individually kick the couple on their backs, and I as therapist was to be the last one to do that. This was a great and dramatic improvisational metaphor in several ways. We kindly and gently kicked them out of therapy and at the same time the nice kicks represented "good luck" to the couple from us all.

Magical stick. When seeing children in therapy sessions the magical stick is fantastic. They enjoy the fantasy and the magic. Adults are often too "grown up" to see these possibilities but presented as a fantasy, it might be acceptable to the couple: "I don't have a magical stick – but let us pretend I have one. I use it here and from now on you live the life together that you both wish. How are you doing as a couple?" (or "What will other people notice?").

Play with time. If we have the idea that our present situation is determined by what has been happening in our childhood, there is no idea of playing with time. What's done is done. If we have the idea of the future and what lies in front of us as influencing our behaviour today, future questions are very constructive. Future questions help people describe their wishes and ambitions, helping them create a narrative of their direction in life. Future questions open up possibilities, as there are no rights or wrongs. There are no ready-made answers and no facts that might disturb the expression of ideas and wishes. It is hard or impossible to dispute what has not yet happened. Future questions can be pointing towards the distant future but also focusing on the immediate future after the session or tomorrow.

I did a consultation with a couple and the man had serious difficulties in imagining what his future would be like. After a while I began talking about what his situation would be like after the session if the afternoon turned out to be like he wished. What would be the differences? How would he and his wife notice? At last, he could begin to describe his preferred afternoon with a lot of details.

Play with position. People are often stuck in their problems and their own feelings. To put yourself in the other person's shoes, switching positions and making this effort can be a new and rewarding experience for both partners. Asking the couple to give advice to other couples is to put them in an expert role and to give the couple a chance to help others (if the therapist asks for permission to pass on their advice to others). An unexpected idea from the therapist is to start the session by asking the couple to interview the therapist. "You know what you want and what important questions you have in mind. Please feel free to ask me what you want".

Sculpting. Many years ago I attended a month-long training with Virginia Satir and was fascinated not only by her as a person but also by the non-verbal way of working with family sculptures. Satir's physical stances (blamer, placater, super-reasonable and distractor) are very useful to demonstrate the relationships in the family without words and the interactional process of three different pictures/sculptures that constitutes the family pattern (Satir, 1976). The positions can't be held for very long time and (you cannot be in the blamer stance or any of the other stances for a very long – you get awfully tired or uncomfortable). The couple can also be asked to create the sculpture themselves. "Make a sculpture of your family without words".

My colleague was more experienced than me around this time and we met a couple. They were worried and anxious since their daughter had some severe eating problems. The daughter didn't attend the session. Suddenly my colleague suggested that the parents make a sculpture of the family. The father reacted immediately and leaned back so suddenly and forcefully that he nearly touched the window. After a while he said "I need a rope." My colleague answered "I'll go and fetch one – just a minute", I didn't know we had a rope in the office, but apparently she knew! When she came back the father took the rope and made a circle with the mother and daughter (as if she had been there) inside and he himself standing outside holding the ends of the rope. He looked satisfied, but the mother was very uncomfortable and said she couldn't stand being locked up in the circle. Sculpting is a strong emotional experience and must of course be handled with care. The parents returned for several sessions, the daughter recovered and the worries of the parents diminished. In couple sessions the partners can be asked to do their sculptures of present relationship and their preferred future sculpture. This can be an emotional and learning experience for the partners. If done in an OAAT session you need to be sure the couple leave the session with ideas and plans of how to continue their relationship work at home.

Metaphors and Fairy Tales. When someone says something like "Don't think of a polar bear!" the immediate reaction for those who hear that is to get the picture of the polar bear in mind. This is natural, normal and how it works. We create a picture of what we experience in interaction with others. The other thing is that pictures tell more than a thousand words as the saying goes. This is why metaphors are so strong and hard to erase or delete. They just stay. Metaphors must be handled with care and timing when expressed in therapy sessions. If they don't fit the couple the metaphors can be destructive, and the couple can react by feeling misunderstood or rejected. If the metaphors fit the couple will have a useful and constructive picture that can be their guiding star. Glass doors and certificate in this chapter is one example of metaphor created collaboratively in the session. There are many more in the book. In Chapters 17 and 18 we present OAAT sessions including how metaphors were created and presented.

A lot of good things are happening in OAAT.

Note

1 Ben Furman is a well-known psychotherapist, trainer and author from Finland.

Chapter 12

An Ordinary Day – OAAT Team, Malmö

Martin Söderquist, Malena Cronholm-Nouicer, Lars Dannerup and Karin Wulff

Brief Stories from Sessions

For several reasons we have chosen to offer couples One at a Time (OAAT) counselling on Tuesdays. It seems like ten OAAT sessions a week fit our service very well. Our service schedules approximately 25–30 new couples a week and the four of us working with OAAT have found it convenient and most concentrated to have all OAAT on the same day. It makes it easier for us to do team sessions and in the breaks between sessions discuss and help each other.

Below follow some examples from OAAT sessions to demonstrate the wide range of problems couples present and the broad palette of hopes and goals they express. There are several examples of different ways of couple – counsellor collaboration. The counsellor seeing the couple is indicated in parentheses. When we began with Single Session Therapy (SST)/OAAT we did follow-ups but currently we don't follow up – we leave the decision to the couple to decide how they want to proceed.

Couple, 35 years old. They schedule a session to discuss their situation. They have tried to have children and been through IVF treatment and assessment for adoption. It has been a difficult and stressful period for them, and they have begun drifting away from each other. During last six months they have been more and more hesitant if they are to continue their relation. Now they have mutually decided they want to continue as a couple and that they need help to communicate in a better way. They tell the counsellor they also have scheduled Traditional counselling.

In the session, both of them say they miss the closeness they used to have. The session focuses on how they can express their needs in a way their partner can accept. There is a shift in the session when they discover they miss and really care about each other. The distance and the conflicts seem to be expressions of misdirected frustration. (Lars).

Couple in their forties. Alice attends the session alone – she couldn't persuade her partner, Roy. They have been a couple for 15 years, and they are socially established with well-paid jobs in a good economy. Alice is hoping the session will help her "get more security and trust in the decision I think I have to make".

DOI: 10.4324/9781003305774-12

Alice and Roy have three children aged five, three and one, and Alice tells the counsellor that a year ago Roy slapped two of the children. Alice talked to pre-school and school, and they made a report to Child Protection, but this report somehow got lost. Some months later the oldest child told the school social worker of the situation with conflicts and quarrels at home, and the school social worker made a new report to Child Protection. Their assessment is completed, and the case is closed without any further measures being taken.

In the session the focus is on Alice's dilemma: separation – or stay with Roy. During the session it is more and more obvious to Alice that she has to make a very hard and difficult decision but the negative consequences of staying with Roy are too huge. Even if she can protect her children, she thinks her health will be damaged, and if so, she won't be able to be there for her children. Alice is on 8–9 on a 1–10 scale as to how sure she is in her decision to separate. Alice expresses her loneliness in this decision, and we talk about support. Who is there for her if she separates? How can she protect herself and her children when she leaves her husband?

Alice tells the counsellor the possibility to have a session within a few days was crucial and very supporting in a situation when she had to make a difficult decision concerning the safety and security of her children. (Malena).

Couple, 55–60 years old. The problem with one of the couple's adult children have stressed their relationship a lot. They have finally decided, after long discussions and much doubt, to schedule a couple session.

The woman tells the counsellor her best hope for the session is that her husband will understand her feelings and her actions. The man wishes they together can find a way to have a calm family life with all their adult children. Both express they want to be supported by their partners.

What they want and what they wish together is in focus the rest of the session. Most of all the necessity for both to know "you are there for me".

The counsellor gives them an exercise to bring home inspired by Karl Tomm (Tomm, personal communication, 2017), The purpose of the exercise is to practice expressing what you want without being interrupted, trying to understand your partner and most of all listen. (Martin).

Couple in their thirties. They have been living together for two years, but at the moment they are living separately. Their child is two years old, and they both have a child from previous relationships, aged five and seven. They decided to live separately because of enormous conflicts with too high level of the conflicts. The woman is very jealous and doesn't trust the man in his relationship to the mother of his child. The man says this is not true at all and say he is falsely and unfairly accused. They both wish to fight less and create a calmer life for the children.

The focus in the session is how they handle conflicts and what they can do individually to stay within the boundaries they themselves are satisfied with. We call this area within the boundaries *tolerance window* (Sicgel, 1999). We focus how they can calm down, how they notice when things are going in the wrong direction and what cause the conflicts. We also talk about decision making, your own responsibility and the importance of doing the right choices for the sake of the children. Before they leave the session the get some printed material of conflict managing. (Karin).

Couples in their thirties. The couple have two children aged three years and eight months. They have scheduled the session because of more and more relationship distance. They have over the years experienced growing stress because of all changes that have pushed them to adjust to new situations like having two children, the move to a new house and owing to the woman´s chronic illness.

They both express a wish for having tools which can help improve their relation. The session focus is how they can "really meet" in everyday life. The man says he has already been thinking of suggesting having a planning meeting every Sunday to make it easier to communicate and collaborate and the woman approve of his idea. Most of all she is glad he is taking this initiative. Together they come up with the suggestion to have a "tea time" to discuss the day every evening when the children are asleep in bed. The counsellor also gives them exercises to bring home like – Daily Checklist, Love Maps and Good Habits. They spontaneously express: "This is what we came here for!" (Lars).

Couple who has been living together for twenty years and having two small children. The process to seek help has been a huge step and they see OAAT as an opportunity to try counselling without a long waiting list. They have been thinking about this for half a year.

Kim is hoping to be more joyful, having more energy and getting a feeling of teaming together with her partner. Sam is hoping to be able to avoid getting into small arguments, get rid of irritation and that they can have feeling of; "It is the two of us, we are a team".

Sam describes his frustration of not being listened to when it comes to small as well as big things. Despite the fact Sam has begged Kim he thinks Kim ignore this. When they have agreed upon a important rule Sam see Kim not living up to their decision. This irritates Sam followed by sarcastic comments and revengeful behaviour from him who have a feeling of not being important to Kim.

Kim describes a feeling of not being equal and a lack of team sense when Sam "jumps in to a situation" when Kim is together with the children. In these instances Kim feels bad, become sad and wants to give up. She tries to go through the day until the children are sleeping. Afterwards the irritation stays with Sam for a long period. They are both very sad and lonely.

We discuss the two important roles – **Parent team** and **Partner team**. When discussing the Parent team, the couple want to focus to allow each other do things in their own way when being individually with the children. They agree everything is fine when one of them isn´t home and they also agree to pick one rule especially important to the children which they want to implement and support each other when they are all together (see Ziegler and Hiller, 2001).

The Partner team is pressured hard – they have gone from two to four in a short period. We discuss how they can protect their couple relationship and make inputs on their emotional account.

They want help with getting closer without talking about problems. The counsellor shows them material they can take home focusing getting to know each other in a new way. The want to have all the pack of cards they can be offered (Love Maps, Sex and Desire, Good Habits) to have something to choose between. (Malena).

Couple, 26 years old. The couple describe their relationship as a constant on and off relationship for four years. At the moment they don't meet very often, and now they need help to decide if they are a couple, just friends or in a poly amorous relation. It becomes evident in the session that the woman would like to be "together" and the man is more doubtful if they can become a "couple".

The conversation in the session is focused on what relationships can be like, what can be expected, what we call different relations and the valuations affecting/ruling us. Another central part of the session is the discussion of how to deal with strong feelings in a relationship when the partners have different views on living together. After the session the couple stay outside the office in the backyard for several hours in a long discussion on their own. (Lars).

Couple 30–40 years old. The couple has been exposed to many challenges last years: health problems, drug abuse, work-related problems, intimate partner abuse and financial difficulties. They have severe difficulties in noticing their partner's efforts in taking care of themselves and can't really trust that the small positive changes they talk about will remain.

The partners have very different views about what they are hoping for, and the counsellor sees their views as totally incompatible. Despite our efforts, we can't get to a common platform for the session, except that both partners want their children to have a good a life as possible. This is strongly confirmed by the counsellor. The recommendation offered to the couple by the counsellor: "Go all in for being parents together – this is crucial for the time being." The couple agree, and they are prepared to do this. The counsellor also suggests that they try, even if it is very, very hard, to put discussions of what has been, their partnership and other things on hold. All things can't be simultaneously done – there is a time for everything. (Martin).

Couple, 35 years old with a little baby. The woman has moved back to the husband after being on her own with the baby for some weeks. She demands relationship changes in order to be able to continue living with the husband. In th past two weeks the man has tried to be calmer and less angry. The woman is willing to give her husband a last chance – the alternative is separation, and she is very determined and clear about this.

They both want a "quarrel-free environment" for the sake of their children but also for themselves, and they are in agreement about the importance of changes that are real changes. They have found a way to avoid conflicts, but this must hold over time. They agree, and both are willing to work hard to do that.

When ending the session, the counsellor tells the couple he is very impressed by the husbands will power to handle the situation and that he really has been listening to his wife, examined himself and is prepared to make a real effort. The counsellor tells the woman he is impressed by her determination, strong will and the fact she is so determined and clear of what she wants and demands. Considering their history of infidelity, quarrels, conflicts, new-born baby and communication problem they have been more successful than they know. The couple is given a "time out" idea, which is building on their own idea proposed in the session and suggestions to observe and focus on every small sign of maturity and good conditions to maintain and continue what they already have done. (Martin).

Parents in their forties. Their daughter is two and a half years old. They didn't plan the pregnancy and the father is from another country. The mother has a chronic disease that decomposes her body and made her totally exhausted the first year or so. She also has a diagnosed case of depression. The father was unfaithful for a period of two years and they scheduled a session when the mother stopped talking to everyone. They both want to communicate better and solve the problem and decide in which country they are to live in. The father wants a loving relationship, but the mother can't imagine this at all.

The focus of the session is how they can structure their communication and they decide the father will move to Sweden at least for a couple of years for the sake of the daughter. The mother decide in the session she can't know at this point what she wants and the father accepts this but at the same time wants do his best to enhance the possibilities for a loving relationship, not just being a parent. (Karin).

Married couple, 35 years old. The couple has two children two and five years old. The woman has for a long time felt an unbalance in their relationship, when it comes to responsibility for children and household. This has affected her feelings, and she is thinking it is too late to do anything about it. The man is feeling unloved, insufficient and powerless. They would like to find their way back to each other, but they are wondering if this is possible.

The session continues with what they long for and if they can consider to slow the process and examine the relationship's possibilities. They decide to give themselves time to work for it and they will use the time to discuss what they want and long for. They both want to meet their partner in her/his needs and wishes. They agree to turn to each other instead of turning inwards or turning towards someone else. The woman says she can't promise her feelings will return, but she will definitively make a try. The counsellor advises them not to evaluate their feelings every day. When it has gone so far that one or both partners think that it is too late, it can take time to get back to the loving feelings, and there is no guarantee that it will happen. (Karin).

Problem couples report when scheduling sessions. The brief stories from sessions above are only small details of all the problems, situations and hopes that couples bring to the session. We see couples in different constellations and with a variety of problems, hopes and goals. Last year we saw more couples with sexual problems, separation-related problems and intimate partner violence. We have also seen more couples with psychiatric diagnosis, either one or both partners. In the Appendix, follow-ups are summarised, and they all have one thing in common: there is no difference in results from SST sessions, no matter what kind of problems clients report.

Many of the couples we see are in individual treatment, one or both partners. It is also common for individual therapists to recommend couple sessions with us when the individual therapy doesn´t give the expected results.

As mentioned earlier, couples choose OAAT for several reasons, and they have many questions and wishes. Questions and problem descriptions like: "Have we done the right things?", "Are we normal?", "How can we handle... .?", "How do we know if/how we are to separate?", "We have decided to separate and we need your advices how to talk to the children!", "We can´t reach each other", "Our feelings are gone", "We just quarrel" and "How do other couples solve problems like ours?". Every couple present their own unique problem description and their unique questions.

There are two special things many couples ask for: Tools and a third-person view of their situation.

Tools are asked for when the couples need to get advice about how to handle their communication, conflicts, relationships and when they need to discuss how to approach a constructive behaviour together. In these cases, the couples and counsellors need to focus and examine the precise nature and purpose of the asked for tools.

The viewpoints of a third person – in this case, the counsellor's reflections on their relationship is often expressed and asked for. The counsellor can respond to this in many ways. The counsellor's questions are not only questions but also presuppositions and influence the session in different directions. "When was the last time you did something together and both of you were content?" is an example of several presuppositions; the couple are actually doing things together, they have done it on several occasions, have experienced events that are good for them, and they want something together.

Another response to the couple with a third-person perspective is to comment how the couple communicate and maybe how they can behave a little bit differently. Example: when your partner says something critical, you can tell her/him "I love you too". A third way to respond is to answer their question, for example: "From what you have told me I think you have done the right things" or "You seem to be quite normal – it is your life situation that is mad/bad".

The question "How do other couple ...?"is legitimate. The way other couples handle and solve problems can give the couple in question valuable thoughts, ideas and hints. Over the years I have collected clients', couples' and families' stories, and with their permission, I tell the couples about some of these stories.

When it comes to make important decisions – these processes are often a long, hard and winding road where what is wished for is blended with or exists parallel with fears. Sometimes I tell couples and families facing important decisions the following:

When my children were small, I, a friend of mine and our children were in a swimming pool. All adults were sitting by the pool side and carefully watching our children. After a while we saw a little girl, 7–8 years old and tiny, climbing the stairs to the upper deck of the jumping tower and I and my friend said to each other: "What is she doing? It is dangerous!". The whole situation turned into a drama. The girl anxiously approached the edge of the deck, 10–12 metres up in the air from the water, looked down and withdraw. She did this several times and gazed at her mother sitting by the pool side. Finally, after at least five to ten minutes, she seemed to have made up her mind what to do and went for it. She made it perfectly, feet first in the water and up she came with arms over her head and a great smile. She and her mother looked at each other and smiled happily. We were not the only ones watching the drama. The whole of the swimming hall rang with applause from all the adults there.

To me, this illustrates how decisions are made. Pros and cons are weighed carefully. How important is this to me? How big is the risk-taking? What support do I have from my network and from the most important person in my life?

The girl in the brief story wanted to do the jump very much, and she did so despite the dangers and fears involved.

OAAT Zoom Sessions with Couples

This section of the chapter is based on the experiences of my couple counsellor colleagues' work in Malmö (Karin W., Malena C-N and Lars D.), of Karl Tomm (Professor of Psychiatry, Faculty of Medicine at the University of Calgary and Director of the Calgary Family Therapy Centre) and of Simon Bloomfields (Swedish family therapist, clinical supervisor and teacher in psychotherapy).

Before the pandemic, most therapy sessions took place in the therapist's office or on home visits. Many therapists, including me, sometimes used letters, telephone and e-mails as a supplement to face-to-face sessions. Video was also used where sessions were videotaped and analysed by the therapist. During the next session the therapist and client/couple/parents looked at the video sequences with focus on supporting communication, attuned behaviour and golden moments (Arts, 1995; Harvey, 1990, 1994; Söderquist, 2002).

We had very limited, if any experience at all, of online therapy.

During the past two years the pandemic has caused a lot of problems in every part of people's lives. All restrictions and lock-downs have forced therapeutic and counselling organisations and teams to find new ways of seeing clients, families and couples.

In this section I will present my colleagues' experiences of the challenges and possibilities of doing therapy and OAAT with couples online.

Challenges and Risks with Online Therapy and SST/OAAT

There are many challenges and risks involved in doing therapy on internet. *The security is not 100%, and violations of confidentiality can be devastating* for the trust between the couple and the therapist. The therapy room as a safe haven is totally lost, if this confidentiality is violated. The problems of internet security and the responsibility to guarantee the appropriate security is not in the hands of therapists – it is the responsibility of technicians, computer programmers and the different providers (Teams, Skype, Zoom). This is why I and many others have been reluctant or at least hesitated to do therapy sessions online. The Family therapy centre in Calgary started with using Zoom but did not trust the security enough and subsequently shifted to Teams. The team in Malmö has also been using Zoom and Teams since the beginning and still do so. Although there have been no security problems so far hackers and ransomware attacks seems to be a threat all the time, not only to companies and local authorities but also to mental health organisations.

Another challenge and risk is the *reduced sense of control* when all you can see and hear is what is on the screen. Poor sound and picture quality or acoustic feedback can destroy the possibility in making the session helpful to the couples. If you don´t hear or see well enough it is hard to really get a grip of what the couple hope for. This needs to be dealt with.

A more severe control challenge is the question of those *who are present* in the session. Are there other people attending but the therapist is unable to see them? Is the session being recorded by someone without a couple – therapist agreement? How are the different situations handled when one of the partners just gets up and leaves the session or if the couple suddenly go offline or if the couple start a physical fight or when discussing sexual problems get aroused and begin with sexual activities? It is impossible to predict what can happen in a therapy session but as mentioned before "Coincidence favours the prepared mind". The therapist can set her/his mind on being prepared for everything but stay focused on the hopes and goals of the couples. The context marking in the beginning of the online session is of utmost importance.

There are more challenges:

People are excluded. Older people might not be used to being online and those people who do not have access to computer are excluded from online therapy. People might be able to borrow a computer but this might not be convenient and can be complicated. If there is free access to computers on libraries, this might be an option but having an online therapy session publicly is not what most people wish. People must have the possibility to have face-to-face sessions within a secure setting.

Reduced sense of personal connection. Less eye contact, a sense of distance when separated by screen and difficulties in noticing small gestures and physical reactions might reduce the personal connection. This can threaten the couple – therapist alliance and collaboration. It is of vital importance to take care with language – words and tone of voice. The therapist needs to be precise, clear and concrete in what is said and done to avoid detrimental mis-understandings. There are less obvious non-verbal signs from the couple to guide the therapist to rephrase, change or modify the questions or reflections.

Therapeutic culture in the team or in the organisation. This can be an obstacle to introducing online therapy as a method of therapy. The culture in the team might define therapy as client and therapist seeing each other in face-to-face sessions and other ways as being less effective, less emotional and inappropriate.

Possibilities and advantages with online therapy.

Logistically there are many advantages with online therapy.

The couples *don't have to travel* to therapists' office and have no parking problems which makes it easier for the couples. They *lose no time* in their stressful everyday lives and can combine the one-hour session with their other activities involving children and work. An obvious advantage is that the partners can *be in different places* and still have the couple session. Business travels, unforeseen traffic problems and sick children and lots of other situations might contribute to cancelled face-to-face sessions but online sessions are possible anyway. For physically challenged (one or both partners) online couple sessions are easily accessible and all the logistical problems for them can be excluded.

Another aspect is that the couples can be in their *safe environment, their homes,* and don't have to go an unknown office where they can be uncomfortable.

Children and adolescents can attend the session but be off screen. Often therapeutic sessions are clearly led by adults with focus on the parents' ideas and suggestions. Therapy sessions are not the primary choice of the children, and they might be reluctant, nervous, defiant and unhappy. The possibility of attending online but off screen makes it easier and more comfortable for the children.

Couples in conflict. If the couple has separated and have to talk about their relationship and need to discuss the children or living arrangements, online therapy is an option. One of the partners might have moved and cannot attend a session in the office of the therapist, or the partners do not want to meet face-to-face due to anger, fear or disgust. With the distance and the screen between them the partners might find it more convenient, and they might be able to handle the situation.

Couples can create a good relationship moment. Couples having the session online in their homes or elsewhere have the opportunity to make something special of the session. They might have babysitting arrangements and made preparations for the session in a number of ways; sitting together apparently cosy on the sofa or in the car and experiencing a good relationship moment when having the couple session.

Therapists have the opportunity to do home visits. When seeing couples in the office the therapist is restricted to the stories the couple tell in the session. Seeing parts of the homes of the couple on the screen gives the therapist a deeper understanding of the couple and an increased sense of what their reality is and the choices they have made for their living. Some couples are proud of their homes, like to be there and show others how they live.

Online therapy opens up for creative ideas. Doing sessions with a reflecting team is of course an option. The couple, therapist, the team and supervisor don´t have to be in the same place – they just need to be online the same time of day. Karl Tomm told me "We have managed to simulate 'reflecting team' work online as well. The team members keep their microphones and cameras off until the reflection when the therapist and clients turn their mic and cameras off. It works reasonably well but is not as rich as the one-way screen system" (Karl Tomm, personal communication). In a Zoom presentation called *From Room to Zoom* for the Swedish Family Therapy Association, Simon Bloomfield suggested some ideas, and I have added some other ideas for couple sessions.

*Break the session down to different parts: 30–40 minutes, break, 30–40 minutes, break, summary and reflections. (After 30–40 minutes in front of a screen you need a break.)

*Doing role play of different kinds. Playing someone else in the family and being interviewed by the therapist or the partner. Externalizing a problem is another option. The therapist interviewing the "anger" or "communication difficulties". A third option is roleplaying the couples are on stage and the therapist is a film director zooming in on small details.

*The partners and the therapist all have the opportunity of being on different screens as a way of creating distance or cooling down if needed to get on in the session.

*Pictures are of course of great use in promoting spontaneity and imagination in therapy, especially given the restrictions of an online based meeting. Drawing a picture on screen can give it more weight.

*Similarly it can be a creative distraction to ask the couples to do something different during the break, for example to each find an object which is older than they are, or to bring to the camera an object they have previously received as a gift from each other or from others. This also helps the couples to think of connections they have to others in the family network.

All of what has been mentioned in previous chapters – inviting couples and open up space for creativity – can be used in online therapy. The difference is that online therapy isn´t as rich, personal and emotional as face-to-face sessions for many couples and therapists.

However, online therapy is still new to the therapy field, and there are probably many more creative solutions to be found.

Bouverie Centre in Melbourne, Australia (www.bouverie.org.au) has developed a great variety of self-paced online courses, streaming services and webinars. Other organisations and teams have also done the same. I am sure that in the future some or much of the therapist training will be online but to license or approve therapists, face-to-face training will be necessary.

Online therapy has most probably come to stay, and the development of therapy models and session formats will continue. It will be a complement to face-to-face sessions offering clients a chance to have therapy sessions easily accessible. I don´t think online therapy will take over the whole field of therapy though. It is probable that a hybrid approach will be the choice for many clients and couples as well as for the therapists and counsellors. Face-to-face sessions will still be the most emotional and intense way of therapy for most couples and therapists.

Chapter 13

OAAT Sessions – Introduction to Full-Length Case Stories

Martin Söderquist

Describing everything going on in a Once at a Time (OAAT) session is very hard. Partly because of the concentration and focus which is not always seen in the text, partly because of how impossible it is to include gestures, mimics and tone of voice that are so vital and important when people interact. In the following descriptions we try to reproduce as much as possible of the session. The four of us writing the chapters from the session room, Chapters 14–18, are in many ways equal – we share different ideas of counselling and therapy, we have been working together for many years and during the past ten years we have created our version of OAAT. At the same time we are different – we are individuals, we have our own therapeutic style and preferences, and we act differently when leading a session. This will be evident in the stories from the session room. The couples are also unique and that makes the sessions similar yet different.

The sessions[1] in the chapters are mainly couple sessions but the format OAAT as mentioned earlier is applicable with clients and families too. Some 80% of the clients at Eastside Family Centre, Canada are individual clients (McElheran, personal communication) and a large proportion of the clients Bouverie Centre, Australia see are families (Young, personal communication).

Note

1 We have omitted all facts that can identify the couples and made some changes to make it even harder to recognise the couples. This is to guarantee absolute confidentiality. In all the chapters we describe what was done in the sessions as accurate as possible.

DOI: 10.4324/9781003305774-13

Chapter 14

Creating Safety and Good Moments

Martin Söderquist

The couple scheduled Traditional counselling and did not choose One at a Time (OAAT) therapy from the beginning. It turned out they attended only one session, in the literature called *unplanned single session* (Talmon, 1990). This is common in all outpatient services as well as in our work with couples.

It is not common when we meet couples that we see rough and very dangerous intimate partner violence. To these couples we recommend to contact the Crisis Centre in Malmö to schedule individual or same sex group (all male or all female) sessions. In recent years we have noticed an increasing number of intimate partner violence in our office. We are not just talking about verbal abuse, threats and violations – we are talking about situations where one or both dangerously cross the boundaries and violates the integrity of the partner. We published an article in the Swedish journal *Socionomen* (Söderquist, Dannerup and Cronholm-Nouicer, 2016) and presented a relationship view on domestic violence inspired by Johnson (2008) and his ideas and research on what he previously called intimate terror and situational violence. According to Johnson situational violence is most prevalent and both partners contribute to the escalation of the conflict and one or both partners cross the partners boundaries by physical assaults/violence.

We presented our model in that article and we call it Possibility Assessment.

In our experience, couple sessions with intimate violent partners are possible and more constructive than is commonly considered in Sweden, at least. The partner, or both, who has crossed the boundaries of the other has to take responsibility for her/his actions and behaviour and the safety for both has to be guaranteed, if seeing the couple together in a session. We are couple counsellor and used to and consequently not reluctant at all to see couples in violent relations, but we are careful to guarantee the safety of both partners. Couple sessions can be very constructive and helpful, but if there are any doubts about serious dangers and safety, the individuals are to be offered individual or group sessions at the Crisis Centre.

Later Johnson changed the concepts to *situational couple violence and coercive controlling violence* – a better way to describe the differences. Johnson also presents two more patterns of partner violence – *violent resistance and*

DOI: 10.4324/9781003305774-14

separation instigated violence. These are not included in our brief and simple model (Johnson, 2008). Reality is not black and white; reality is varied in many different ways, and we see our model as a good enough map to orient yourself when seeing a intimate partner violence couple.

Coercive Controlling Violence	Situational Couple Violence
Unilateral. Continued and Controlling Power	Bilateral. Problem of Losing Control
"High Level Violence". Great risk of children in danger/seriously affected. Great risk of serious danger / death for the victim	"Low Level Violence". Children in danger of being witness. Risk of danger for both
Abuse and addiction, Psychiatric problems and Criminality	Lesser degree of abuse and addiction, Psychiatric problems and Criminality
Fear and danger rules the relation, Question of time when next violent situation occurs, the victim has no power in the situation	Some uncertainty and discomfort but the victim / both partners have power in the relation. Both partners feel secure enough in their situation
Excuses, denial and minimizing of violence	The most active in violent behavior / both partners take full responsibility for their own behavior. Some degree of excuses and minimizing
The offender is not ready to do anything and make demands on the victim to do all changes in behavior.	The most active in violent behavior / both partners are ready to try to make necessary changes to make the relation safe for both.
One partner wants the violence to stop/ separate, the other wants the relation to continue whatever costs.	Both agree on continuing the relation and want a future together.
Separation = Danger. It is not possible to talk about separation, Serious danger.	Separation = Possibility. It is possible and OK to talk about separation.
What goes on in family is kept secret for other people, no one knows and children are affected / also abused.	People outside the family knows about what is going on and can be of help.
Latent, subtile and threatening body language and gestures are very hard for others to observe.	Latent, subtile and threatening body language and gestures are absent or more easily observable for others.
The therapist/counsellor has a feeling of danger, threat and severe risk.	The therapist / counsellor has a feeling of enough safety and possibilities.
INDIVIDUAL SESSIONS ARE RECOMMENDED. WHEN CHANGES ARE MADE AND SAFETY IS GUARANTEED – CONCURRENT PARTNER SESSIONS / COUPLE SESSIONS.	COUPLE SESSIONS ARE RECOMMENDED AND IS A POSSIBILITY TO HANDLE CONFLICTS AND ENHANCE THE RELATION.

Figure 14.1 Possibility Assessment

When seeing these couples we are inspired by Wade (1997), Jenkins (1990), Stith et al. (2011), Hamel (2007; 2008), Groen and van Lawick (2009) and Gottman (see Bradey et al., 2011). I and a colleague of mine in Helsingborg wrote a chapter in Hamels book *Intimate partner and family abuse* (2008) on our sessions with a mother and her teenage son.

The excerpt that follows show the difficulties when seeing a couple in a violent relationship:

Allan Wade[1] attended, in the session room, one of my couple sessions as part of a reflecting team. His first reflection after a while was a question: "How come you asked the woman first about what had happened?" Unfortunately I couldn't give a reasonable explanation to him or the couple.

After the session I was thinking that all our behaviours aren't always thoroughly planned, but all our behaviour has consequences. If one half of the couple was defined as being coercive or controlling, my question to the woman could have been catastrophic. Asking the woman to describe what the man had done to her would have been to take a stance against her and allow the man to be free from responsibility. If he were to give his version after the woman, he could just "correct" her version.

If, however, the couple were defined as situational violent and both were involved in escalating the conflict, it wouldn't be so important who was to start telling their stories. As long as both versions are free to express and listened to. If one of the partners is more active and pushing he or she is to be asked first and by that take his/her responsibility.

The following case illustrates a session in which couple violence can be called situational partner violence.

Maxi called us and wanted to schedule an appointment, after being recommended by several persons' friends as well as the authorities. Maxi doesn't say so much over the phone, but my colleague decides to schedule a couple session with us and recommends Maxi to schedule an individual appointment with the Crisis Centre.

Maxi and Kim begin the session by telling the counsellor (Martin Söderquist) that their fights and conflicts have escalated and become worse over the last couple of weeks. They both know how to provoke each other which leads to verbal assaults and violence, physical fights and blows. The fight that resulted in the phone call to us ended in hard pushes, Maxi wrestled down and hit Kim while lying on the floor. Maxi somehow stopped from hitting Kim a second/third time and left the room. All the noise and shouting worried the neighbours, and they made a phone call to the police. The police came in a few minutes and the whole situation calmed down. The couple have a small child who was sleeping. If she/he heard or saw anything was not clear.

We go through the whole situation in details, how they both experienced and how they could see afterwards what they had done, especially their behaviour during the fight. They both felt misunderstood and unfairly accused, and when one of them smiled and didn't understand what they were talking about, the partner saw the smile as something heavily derogatory. They both provoked each other in the extreme when they reacted as they did. A push led to a struggle, and in the worst-case scenario this could have ended in dangerous violence and a disaster for them and their child.

The theme for the session continues with how certain they are these situations will never again be part of their life. On a scale of 1–10 they both are convinced they are at 7–8, where 10 stands for physical aggression that will never happen again. As counsellor, you will never cease to be surprised. Both were high on the scale, and from what had been said so far in the session, I didn't expect these numbers.

When we continue the session Kim and Maxi have several ideas about to what and how they can do to create safety in their relation. They mention for example they can leave the room, decide to fight only in a certain room (not the bedroom) or take a walk outside to calm down. After having done this they can start over in a calmer way. Kim is very decisive and firm in never accepting any violence from now on, and Maxi says: "I will never behave like this again". The day before the session they dealt with a potentially dangerous situation and avoided a risky fight. They cooled down in a way they hadn't managed before by reminding themselves of the dangerous fight had got them to schedule a couple session. Neither of them was willing to go through a situation like that again and they were also thinking ahead to the couple session a few days later. What helped them most of all was thinking of their child and the importance of their parental protection.

Maxi and Kim are somewhat hesitant when I asked them "What tell you these violent and dangerous situations will never come up again?". Maxi says they have to work hard to try to understand each other and seek help from others. Kim has some difficulties in expressing but is used to manage things and is convinced of the coping possibilities now. Earlier in the session Kim said "I won't accept violence"; if there is violence again Kim will leave, and this is expressed with much emphasis and strength. This is not unusual for persons being abused to say, but Kim's determination is so strong that the two of us listening to Kim have no reason to doubt her.

The session ends with a brief "individual reflection time" (I leave the room for a few minutes) to go through the session on my own. This is necessary to gather my thoughts, think the session through, decide what to reflect to the couple and what to suggest them. When coming to difficult problems and intensive sessions this is especially important.

I begin my reflections to the couple by saying: "I asked you what tell you how you will manage to avoid potentially situations from now on" and then I continue: "I want to tell you what I have noticed which seems to be very important to you":

- You talk about your conflicts and fights last weeks openly
- You are aware of your own behavior and your part of what happened that was too much for both

- You take individual responsibility for what you said and did when everything went too far and you don't blame your partner
- Yesterday you found a strategy to calm down and managed the situation in a good way
- You are prepared to and you have plans to secure safety for all three in the family
- Your little child is most important of all and you want your child to have a safe childhood.
- My suggestion is; Keep on observing what you do yourself and what your partner does to contribute to safety in the family".

We agree to schedule another session. A week later, before next session, Maxi calls me and tells Kim say they don't need the session. Maxi tell me everything has been calm and Maxi agree with Kim – they don't need sessions.

I tell Maxi they are always welcome to return – "the door is always open".

Telephone follow up one year later.

Maxi and Kim are still a couple and say they have managed to avoid all potential dangerous situations despite all the challenges and stresses they have been exposed to. They both have found ways to calm down and leave potentional negative situations. Most of all they have had good and positive moments together they very much have appreciated. They tell about their last vacation and some other good moments the two of them and all three together enjoyed.

My reflections:

The one session with Kim and Maxi focused on how to handle conflicts and creating safety. First of all it was important to lower the level of conflict and help the couple deescalate. Secondly, not so focused in session, building on the positive and good in their relationship. What most of all convinced me; they took personally responsibility, were prepared to do their best to avoid fights and they managed a potentially dangerous situation the day before the session. They were also very realistic and open with their worries and doubts, I saw it as a good sign, but Kim was hesitant. In the session Kim mentioned being used to handle things and having self-confidence, but... . To me there were some remaining questions after the session: Were their plans concrete and detailed enough if they ended up in a real difficult situation? How strong did they want to remain as a couple?

There was only one session. They showed me and convinced themselves they had enough individual and mutual strategies to manage their family life including creating good and fantastic moments together. This was something they both wanted and could manage together.

Note

1 Allan Wade from Vancouver Island in Canada is known for his work with clients faced with oppression and violence and for his definition of violence as a natural and normal response to oppression and violence. His model is called *response-based therapy.*

Chapter 15

To Know Your Way About[1]

Lars Dannerup

Virginia Satir is known to have said; to have one choice is no choice; to have two choices is a dilemma; and to have three choices offers new possibilities.

A key concept in our work with One at a Time (OAAT) therapy is the predefined, and limited, time given to each couple. It follows that even if the couple express that they don't know how to move on together, and hence sought our counsel, it is essential to swiftly establish their desired direction of the session.

One perspective of counselling is that we can help couples to formulate a direction that they can move towards, and to identify goalposts that signal that they are on the right track. Crucially, we can assist them in realising that they are already on the right track, and, perhaps most importantly, how they made that possible.

It is common that a couple in the beginning of a session have multiple, and sometimes conflicting, goals and hopes linked to what they want to achieve in the session. Sometimes a couple is in agreement about the best possible outcome, while another couple might disagree on why they even made the appointment in the first place.

In one of his lectures, John Gottman stated that one of the most important measurements to monitor is where in the relation to what he called the higher level and the lower level on which a couple finds itself.

In every relationship, different needs must be met. While the needs can vary from couple to couple, most can be addressed by answering questions such as: *Do you know what I need?* and *Are you there for me?* The avenues in which these questions are addressed also vary, but often include emotional conversations, during the exercise of shared activities or physical closeness and sex, or when talking about the future. The higher level of a relationship is attained when each individual perceives that the frequency, quality and outcome of these conversations are adequate to meet their needs. The lower level measures how a couple manages conflicts and disagreements. Should the level of conflict be too vicious, or if conflicts repeatedly result in deadlocks, then the lower level of the relationship is at such a low that it presents a tangible threat to its continuation. Furthermore, even if the higher level is satisfactory,

DOI: 10.4324/9781003305774-15

it does not offer a bulletproof protection against too much conflict. When a relationship is characterised by conflict and disagreement, it gets too cumbersome to entertain, the rift between the individuals expands, and they cease investing in the relationship. At this stage, the higher level and the lower level are no longer in play. Rather, the players have left the field and lean towards quitting the relationship.

When talking with a couple about how to attain, or sustain, a higher level of a relationship the focus often is on how to strengthen togetherness and manifest attention for each other's needs. Reversely, what comes to the fore when discussing the lower level is often patterns of conflict, how to break a negative trajectory, and instead boost the relationship to a higher level. Beyond these frameworks, questions about separation occurs when there is no engagement left to uphold the relationship or no intention to participate in reaching for a higher level.

This perspective can be a useful tool for both counsellors and couples to rapidly establish the focus of the OAAT: maintaining or strengthening an already high level of the relationship, changing a low-level relationship to a higher level, or ending the relationship.

Eva and Eric had made an appointment for OAAT. It was Eric that had made the call a couple of weeks ago and on the phone they both had stated the urgency of an OAAT session which suited them well. Now they were both seated in front of me and waited for the session to start. It was the first time they had sought counselling, and like most first-time couples they were a bit uneasy about what was to come. After noting down the usual statistical information, and commenting on the weather, it was raining cats and dogs, and they were both wet from the downpour, I ask:

LARS: What could happen in this session that would make it worthwhile for you coming here today?

They look at each other, and

ERIC: You go first.
EVA: The autumn has been really challenging. We can hardly look at each other without getting annoyed, and it doesn't take much for us to start an argument. The smallest thing can trigger a row that goes on for hours. Sometimes I really lose my temper, but strangely enough the situation has improved slightly since Eric set up this appointment.
ERIC: Yeah, you are right about that. Our relationship hasn't been this good in several months. However, this weekend we probably had the worst conflict that we have ever had. We came really close to ending the relationship this time.
EVA: It can't go on like this. We can't continue to hurt each other this way, something has to change. We need to acquire tools that can help us to avoid getting in to these fights.

LARS: So, from what I gather is that if we had met before this weekend, you would mostly have had good things to say about your relationship and the way things were going.

EVA: Yes, yes indeed. But this weekend was terrible.

She glances over at Eric, and continues:

EVA: You said that you could not go on. That it was impossible to live with me. You cried and cried. I really thought you would leave me.

LARS: I understand that this weekend was really challenging, it sounds like it was a really tough situation for both of you. Is it alright if we get back to that in a moment? Because before that, I would like to know more about what was happening that made you feel that things were going in a good direction the past weeks. Was there anything in particular that you appreciated in one another?

Comment: In OAAT, like in any other session, we constantly value what questions to ask. The questions we posit determines which directions the session takes. During the first minutes of the session, each of three directions are available for us to focus on: the higher level, the lower level, or the end station. According to the couple, the past weeks have been a marked improvement in their relationship which could indicate that they have made improvements on the higher level. On the other hand, the conflict during the weekend was so bad that the lower level clearly posed a threat to their relationship. Eric had even articulated that he couldn't stand the situation anymore, that he wanted to end it. If we as counsellors are uncertain about which direction to take, we often start by exploring the higher level, anchored in the notion that it is conducive to build on what is already working well

ERIC: There was more calm, a different sort of harmony between us.

LARS: More calm, increased harmony. Could you mention how you thought Eva contributed to the improved environment.

ERIC: Well, yes. There was this one occasion when we were out for a walk. The weather was nice, things felt fine between us, and we were even holding hands. Then she started talking about everything that needed to be done when we got back home; the house needed tidying and the shopping had to be done. Things that she typically rants about. Consequently, I felt how I got more withdrawn, and my mood deteriorated. I let go your hand and expected that you would get cranky with me.

Eric looks at Eva:

ERIC: Then you stopped suddenly, took my hand, looked me in the eyes and said "I'm sorry. Here I go again talking about trivial things instead of enjoying the moment. I guess I am not always so easy to live with..."

Eric goes quiet for a moment.

LARS: Tell me more about why this moment was important to you.

ERIC: To be honest. I think this was the first time that I ever heard Eva apologise for anything. But more importantly, I felt that she cared about me, that she liked to be with me.

LARS: It sounds like it was something that you really appreciated. How do you think Eva noticed it?

ERIC: I'm not sure.

"Did you notice it Eva?", he asks her with a glance.

EVA: Yes I did (to Eric with a smile). You said that it was alright, and smiled at me. You didn't go down the path about how irritating I was, but left it at that. Then we continued the walk in a good atmosphere. I have given some thought to the fact that I get angry so quickly, especially when I feel stressed. I am aware that that is frustrating for you, Eric.

LARS: It sounds like you have given some serious thoughts about your own behaviour. What made you stop and apologise to Eric?

EVA: I don't know really,... it just, well,... One thing that has been helpful lately is that Eric has asked much more about me, how I am doing... You know, it has been a lot recently, with all the quarrels, and then he gets withdrawn.

LARS: If we now move to the argument you had this weekend, was it something different this time compared to previous conflicts.

ERIC: I don't think so. I was really upset. You were raging and just kept on shouting. I just felt really exhausted and shut down.

EVA: I don't think I ever seen you this upset (starts to sob).

LARS: Would you like to share what is in those tears.

EVA: I get really frustrated when you shut down (while looking at Eric) You withdraw, and it feels like you have given up on us and don't care what happens next. Do you realise how horrible that feels? I feel totally alone, and then I get really mad, really really mad.

LARS: So, you feel alone and abandoned, and the result is anger? It sounds to me like when the both of you are in a conflict, one expresses anger and the other shuts down, which further deepens the conflicting positions and escalate the situation.

EVA: Yes, that is exactly it. And I also get afraid that you will leave me, she says and continues to sob.

LARS: What do you hear Eva saying?

ERIC: She feels angry, alone, and afraid that I will leave her.

LARS: And what does that make you feel?

ERIC: Well, I actually feel... a bit happy about it (chuckles).

Eva stops her sobbing and looks at him.

LARS: Happy?

ERIC: Yes. Because maybe it isn't so bad when Eva gets angry.

LARS: How do you mean?

ERIC: If she at the same time is afraid that I will leave her, then that must mean that I am important to her. I am not just miserable to be with.

LARS: So perhaps it is the anger that tells you that you are miserable as a partner.

ERIC: Yes, indeed. That's when I shut down, but if I don't do that, there might be a way forward...

LARS: There might be a way forward.

Comment: We continue the session by discussing the elements of their conflict pattern; what thoughts and feelings did the row during the weekend spark? What triggered their anger, and what made Eric retreat to his bubble. At the end of the session I asked them what had been useful and what they could do differently next time they recognised that they were approaching a conflict, Eva stated: "It was really important for me to be made aware of how happy it made Eric feel when he realised that I was afraid of losing him. I guess that is not so easy to understand when I get upset, so I will make an effort to get better at telling him how important he is to me". To this, Eric responded: "I need to proactively share that I am entering my bubble, and that we need to break the pattern which is likely to lead to a conflict. Maybe just taking a break or doing something completely different".

In a session, there is always something that we as counsellors could have done differently. We could have asked more about a particular issue or gone more into depth into one part of the discussion, or maybe even avoided to ask about something that we in fact did ask about. So, what thought processes can help us to understand if what we have achieved during a session has been adequate? Our aspiration is that OAAT will lead to some sort of change in the behaviour of the couple we meet. The couples we see often mention that they want tools, new perspectives, or guidance to change the situation in which they currently find themselves. From our position as counsellors, we therefore hope that the couple will leave the room with a more effective toolbox compared to the one they had before the session. This tool can be a new thought, a new feeling, or an idea of how to improve the relationship. Ultimately, we want to offer the couple a roadmap that stakes out a promising direction forward, or one that makes them confident to follow the path that they have already embarked upon. The signpost we are looking for is a line that are built on the couple's resources and what they have already embarked upon - all done in one session.

Note

1 A brief version of this chapter is published in Söderquist, 2018.

Chapter 16

Team and Progress

Karin Wulff

Imagine a situation where you are going to prepare dinner without knowing what you have at home. You know you'll make something edible, and you know when it's ready. But you know nothing about the content. This is how it is to work with One at a Time (OAAT) therapy.

Session with Team

The team meets a quarter of an hour before the scheduled session. It is decided who will lead the session and who will follow the session behind a screen. The session is not recorded, and the team is not able to call in a message during the session to the counsellor. The couple has already received information at the time of scheduling that we work with team, so it is a conscious choice they make. After an hour of the session, the couple counsellor takes a break to discuss with the rest of the team for about ten minutes. The discussion in the team is summarised to be presented to the couple. During this time, the couple is given the task of thinking about what in the conversation they have benefited from. After the session, the person who lead the session receives feedback from their colleagues.

This form of conversation is very resource-intensive, and we therefore only have one team session every two weeks. The purpose of team sessions is above all to maintain a high quality through openness and to develop the format of OAAT. This is shown in the following case.

Today we agree that I will lead the session. We share the information we have about the couple.

Klara and Adrian are married and in their 40s. They have been together for ten years and have two children, Sara three years old and Samuel four months old. The couple represents our most common target group: about a third of those who schedule couple counselling are 30–40 years old and have children aged 0–6 years. It is a week since Klara and Adrian scheduled the session. They tell me that they also have scheduled a session for traditional couple counselling in two to three months.

DOI: 10.4324/9781003305774-16

The team asks of my ideas before the session. I answer that I want to carefully examine what Klara and Adrian have already done that are in line with their goals, and that I want to try not to take for granted that I know what the problem is and what it is due to, or signal that I would know what the solution is. I want to create a calm setting for me and them in which we together can explore what could help them further towards what they want.

I give the team the task of affirming the couple's challenges as well as abilities, actions and reasoning that seem to be helpful to them. I also want the team to have ideas of advice and good ideas to the couple if that is what the couple wants.

The team asks what I want them to observe when it comes to my efforts. I want them to notice what the balance between my management and my compliance looks like and how well I let my questions follow their answers.

We talk about the fact that the couple also has scheduled a session of traditional family counselling. Would it be possible to introduce the idea that one conversation might suffice? We agree that I should keep it in the back of my mind and express if it is relevant.

The first encounter. We sometimes say that as it begins, it usually ends. This means that the first encounter is of great importance, and therefore I do my best to directly create a good contact. I'm the one who opens the door when they get here. I am thinking of small details such as calm, warmth, eye contact, handshakes and fair distribution of attention. I ask if they want to meet the team that will help us today and they want to do that.

The session. I start by informing Klara and Adrian about our confidentiality, that we will take a break for team discussion after an hour, that I will talk to the team and come back with a summary, that they have the opportunity to schedule a new session, their own decision and their assessment if they wish to do so. They get the opportunity to ask questions about me, the session and couple counselling.

I tell what I know about them, which is not much, and I mention that I want to know a little about how come they contacted us and something about what they want to see as a result of the session. I want to listen to them one at a time as their wishes and experiences may be different. They can start where they want. I ask if it's an okay way for them to start, and they think so.

The couple talks about experiences of several miscarriages, IVF attempts and breastfeeding every two hours. They are both completely exhausted emotionally as well as physically. Klara experiences a strong sense of injustice and loneliness. Adrian feels powerless and inadequate in Klara's eyes. Both feel that they are no longer kind to each other. Two weeks ago, it came to a point when Adrian in a conflict expressed that he "gives up the relationship".

In the session, Adrian says that "it was something I said in affection, it is not what I want, I want us to find our way back to each other, that we are a little kinder and more open to each other, that we talk more". Klara concludes with a tired smile: "We are so fragile. I wish we had 36 hours in one day".

I make an attempt to affirm their difficulties and normalise their situation by describing that life's challenges create stress and lack of sleep. We become more fragile. When we are not in such good shape, it is more difficult to be who you want to be, and this often leads to conflicts and a feeling of distance and loneliness.

Changes already made. Early in the conversation, I want to examine changes already made. The purpose is to highlight the couple's own abilities, strengthen their sense of being able to influence the situation and from a relational perspective show how their behaviour makes a difference for themselves and each other. Highlighting the progress already made is in line with my approach. The couple are experts on their lives, and change takes place mainly between sessions and not during sessions. My role is to create the opportunities to talk about what is happening in a constructive way. My starting point is that people are constantly trying to handle situations and difficulties based on their conditions. I therefore assume that they have done something to try to change their difficult situation for the better. In a challenging and stressful situation, it is more difficult for us to see what is positive. Questions about changes already made help the couple to see their progress. To build a platform that the couple can start from to move on to the next step, I try to deepen and strengthen what the couple describes. I do this by asking the couple what difference the made progress does to them and what it means to them.

In today's session, the couple mentions that their situation has improved a bit recently. I choose to focus on it for most of the session. Here is a short excerpt from the session that shows how I try to focus what the couple has already accomplished:

KARIN: You mentioned that something has gotten a little better. What do you think you have done that is in line with what you want?

ADRIAN: We have thought more about each other, the tone has been more relaxed. Klara has asked "Could you do that?" instead of saying "We have to do".

KARIN: Is there anything special Klara has done that has been important to you? I think of small things, no big gestures.

ADRIAN: Yes, she has asked how it was at work.

KARIN: What difference does it make for you?

ADRIAN: Then it feels like I also exist. That it's not just about taking care of Samuel when I get home, but that I also mean something.

KARIN: What else has Klara done that has been important to you?

ADRIAN: She has asked: "Could you?" instead of saying "We have to", the tone has been more relaxed. It is important how you say things and in what tone.

KARIN: Is there anything special that Adrian has done that has been important to you?

KLARA: Yes, he is more aware of how I feel. When I was breastfeeding, he came up and caressed me.

KARIN: What difference does it make for you?

KLARA: I feel that he is caring, he takes care of me and shows that he understands that it is difficult (She breastfeeds every two hours and has painful milk congestion). He pays attention to how I feel.

KARIN: What else has Adrian done that is in line with what you want and need?

KLARA: He makes an effort to get home from work early. I know it's hard for him, but he's trying. He also suggests that I go to bed and rest.

When it feels like the progress already made is sufficiently explored and the session begins to come to an end, I start to think more in the direction of the future about what could be the next step for the couple. In the phase of life they are in, of course, most of the energy goes to parenthood, and the relationship may be left behind. I therefore ask if there has been something in their relationship before that they are missing now or would like a little more of. "Adventure, it's not so much adventure now," says Adrian with a smile. I confirm that it can really be a feeling you long for and ask if there is something small, small, they could do in this situation that would still give a glimpse of a sense of adventure. "We could have lunch outside", Klara suggests. "Yes, just something that is outside the home and not at the Supermarket," says Adrian. "We could take a walk," he then suggests.

It is now time to take a short break and talk to the team. The couple is asked if there is anything special they want from my colleagues. They have no special wishes but say it will be exciting to hear what they have to say.

Sometimes in situations like this we suggest the couple during the break to think about what they found useful from the session, i.e. if there is something special that has been helpful. You can do this to reinforce something that seems to work well or as a support when you feel unsure about whether or what has been helpful. When we suggest this, we always begin the summary by hearing how they reasoned during the break. The summary of the team and the couple counsellor can then be included in the couple's experience.

Talk to the team during the break. The break is seven to ten minutes long. When I meet the team, I first get a brief encouraging comment about the work I have done. A colleague says, for example, that I did a good job that stayed and deepened the couple's already made progress. Then I get the question what I want now. What happens during the session sometimes or often changes what the counsellor thought before the session. The question from the team makes it possible to change the order. This time, however, I have no need to change my order, and the team is invited to speak freely, albeit one at a time, based on what they think is important that I convey. I want them to confirm the couple's experience of their situation, give them positive feedback on what they have accomplished and suggest something that could be an appropriate next step. Here I mainly have a listening position and ask only one or two clarifying questions while I write down what I find useful. The person leading the session always has the right to determine the design of the summary. It happens, of course, that we as a team have different ideas. If, as a session leader, I do not feel completely comfortable presenting an idea, while at the same time I think the couple could benefit from it, I say that one of my colleagues thought or suggested one or the other.

Summary. When I return to the couple (it is always the session leader who leaves the room during the break), I begin with a short context marking. For example, it could be that I say: "Now I and the team have gathered our thoughts and ideas that we want to share with you". If the couple has been given a task during the break, I start by hearing of their thoughts about the task they were given. The most common task is for them to think about what they benefited from during the session. This is the summary that the couple received from me:

"You have really been through a lot: IVF treatments, miscarriages and now Samuel who wants to breastfeed all the time and is not as happy as Sara was when she was little. It has taken a lot of energy for a long time, and it is within that context you must handle your situation today. That is tough and has made you both fragile."

"This is what happens so beautifully: One of you signals that 'this is not how we can have it', and you respond to that invitation! That's exactly what needs to be in relationships."

"In a short time you have started to turn the ship in the right direction! In the last week alone, you have done several small important things that make a big difference. You, Adrian, caressed Klara when she was breastfeeding, tried to get home earlier from work and suggested to Klara that she go and rest for a while. You show that you care and understand how Klara feels. You, Klara, have asked Adrian how his day has been, you have asked if he 'could' do something instead of saying 'we have to', and you have used a kinder tone."

"You have also thought about effort and effect. It is wise to look at it when energy levels are low, and it is difficult to find time for recovery. You have concluded that lunch and a walk could be just right now when it comes to effort and effect. In line with the fact that you are already kinder and more open to each other, we would like to suggest that you continue to notice when your partner does something that you appreciate and give each other positive verbal feedback. It makes a difference to express in words what you appreciate. A detail is a small thing that makes a big difference."

Adrian and Klara listen attentively to the summary. Adrian takes Klara's hand when I give examples of what they have already done for each other.

The conversation ends with me saying: "It was nice to meet you and you are always welcome to book a new appointment. It could be next week, in six months or in three years".

Team discussion after the session. After the session, we sit in the team for ten minutes and the person who lead the session could reflect upon the session. After that, the team gives feedback. We do it in a structured format that we call two green and one yellow. This means that each team member says two things that the session leader has done well and present one idea about another choice that could have been made in the session.

For example, a colleague thought it was good that I gave the couple the opportunity to choose if they wanted to start telling something about reasons for scheduling the session or something about what they hoped the session would lead to. Another colleague thought it was nice that I picked up that they mentioned early in the session that something had gotten a little better and that I delved deeper into it. One of the yellow comments was that I could have taken note of their description that they were a little more "kind and open" and explored it more.

Reflections

By exploring changes already made, it is often possible to help the couple forward during a single conversation. My experience is that people almost without exception do something to try to change and deal with a difficult situation. Questions about what they have already done show my confidence in their ability to influence and change. It helps to create hope, which is helpful as couples usually seeks help when they experience that the situation is difficult. By building on what is happening, good circumstances are co-created to find a suitable next step. Despite the limited information that the counsellor has access to before the session, the team can together create a comprehensive summary and come up with ideas and suggestions that are in line with the couple's hopes and possibilities. Teamwork provides security and contributes to learning. It makes it possible to capture more perspectives that are important to the couple. The structure also provides a pleasant framework for everyone, and within it, creativity can be given more space. It gets better, and it´s more fun.

Chapter 17

Stories and Fairytales as an Opportunity in OAAT

Malena Cronholm-Nouicer

Fairy tales, pictures and metaphors are often very useful in sessions, as a way to express a lot in a short period of time. Images and metaphors can be very influential, but also an excellent way to express understanding, affirmations and show opportunities. This is a description of a session I had with a couple:

Sonya and Adam schedule One at a Time (OAAT) therapy in a situation where they are worried about how the couple relationship has developed in recent years. They want to try if family counselling can be something for them and therefore choose to schedule OAAT and get an appointment in a couple of days.

The couple, who are in their forties, first met 11 years ago after they had been actively seeking a partner for love and family formation for a longer time. They quickly decided to "go for it". They have been a couple for several years and have three children, four, seven and nine years old. They are both careful to point out that they are sure that they want to live together but that they want more out of the relationship. The couple describes that the relationship has gradually deteriorated and that there is now most often irritation, anger and a feeling of distance between them. I wonder what it is that makes them seek family counselling right now. The couple describes that they managed to have a conversation with each other after one of many quarrels and together they decided that "we cannot have it like this!" They share a concern that their love might end in the long term, if there is no change. I further ask about how they would notice that the session here today would be helpful and how the couple relationship would then start to proceed in the right direction. Adam describes that he would feel more joy and a sense of closeness. Sonya says that she would feel calmer, less irritated and have a sense of meaning. They say that they would like to be more relaxed in each other's company and in the family, laugh more and feel joy for life and each other. Sonya describes that she often feels annoyed and describes that she has a hard time really understanding why. She might have outbursts of anger against Adam who feels attacked. He, in turn, is disappointed by Sonya's angry and irritated tone and withdraws. Life consists of routines and being able to keep up with what they have on the "to do" list. Sonya describes a

DOI: 10.4324/9781003305774-17

strong feeling of inadequacy and stress where the irritation becomes an expression of this. Adam describes that he "bites together" and does not understand that Sonya still has feelings of love for him when she gets so angry. Adam is the one who decides on things and goes in to repair and fix the house to make it good and comfortable for the family.

Adam's original family, parents and two siblings, live abroad, and Sonya only has her father left alive who has alcohol problems. Sonya and her sister have some contact by phone, but they rarely meet as she lives 80 km away. This means that Sonya and Adam do not have a natural person to ask for help with, for example, childcare, which means that they can feel lonely. "We have to manage this," is Adam's approach. "How are we going to handle this" is Sonya's question.

Everyday life is filled with "musts" and both feel that there is hardly any energy left for themselves. In the evenings when the children go to bed, they do things in different places, Sonya prepares for the next day and Adam goes up to the attic to continue the renovation of the house. Sonya feels that she takes care of all the logistics and does a lot of work that isn't visible. Adam focuses on rebuilding the attic in order to eventually be able to offer the children their own room. He wants it to be safely built and beautiful, so he has full focus while Sonya feels that he is in his own bubble.

The couple also mentions that their sex life right now is non-existent. Sonya takes the initiative and wants to have sex with Adam, but he withdraws and does not feel access to his desire which becomes a vicious spiral of guilt and shame in both of them. They share feelings of being "not ok", not being loved and appreciated, and Adam describes that desire is affected by the criticism he feels.

We start talking about what they think a good relationship really contains. When it turns out that both Sonya and Adam are interested in good food, I ask if a couple relationship could be compared to a really good soup, where the base is a tasty broth. We remind each other of the story "cooking soup on a nail". In the fairytale, the good soup was apparently cooked on a nail, but the soup was in fact very juicy and tasty not only from the nail but from all the small but important ingredients that were actually boiled with it. What is needed for the couple relationship to become such a really good, tasty couple broth? We're talking about what exactly their pair broth should contain. We talk about the need to protect their relationship on a daily basis by, for example, taking time for a short moment to listen with interest how the partner is doing. To go to bed together, they also agree feels important right now. They also need to give each other appreciative, encouraging and affirmative comments in everyday life.

The couple looks happier and lighter when we talk but they raise concerns. How should the time be enough for everything? Children, work, housework, friends, leisure activities, etcetera. There is so much that is nice, but many "musts" take over.

I ask if I can tell them a story that I have come to think of (inspired by Grete Bruun, a Danish psychotherapist). The couple nods. It is the story of the students who asked their experienced teacher and lecturer about the meaning of life.

STUDENTS: But tell us. What is the meaning of life?
TEACHER: Hmm, how should I try to describe it … I think I do like this… I show you instead of talking so much…

The teacher then takes out a glass jar and carefully fills it with large stones. "Is the glass jar full now?" the teacher then the students ask.

TEACHER: Yes, it looks like that.

Then the teacher takes pebbles and puts them in the jar that falls down between the large stones.

TEACHER: Is the jar full now?

The students laugh:

STUDENTS: Yes, now the jar is full!

Then the teacher takes a handful of sand and lets it seep into the jar. It goes in pretty much.

STUDENTS: Ahaa, it is clear that the sand that is so fine-grained also fit. But what do you mean by this? We asked you about the meaning of life!
TEACHER: Yes, I think that the big stones are what is really important in life, which gives us meaning. These are our important relationships, the ones we like a lot and want to surround ourselves with. The pebbles are perhaps our job we go to, the one that matters but is not as important. The sand is all that other… rubbish…

The students look and ponder.

TEACHER: But what happens if we pour on the sand first?

The teacher takes another glass jar and pours sand up to the edge of the jar. -Then there is only room for....sand.
The teacher takes the first jar which is filled with large and small stones and sand. He is now pouring into the cup of tea he just brewed. The tea seeps into the sand with ease.

TEACHER: With this jar, there is also always room for a cup of tea together!

Sonya and Adam look at each other. Sonya's eyes fill with tears and Adam takes her hands. Life is short, Adam whispers and Sonya nods. Adam reminds Sonya of their friend who worked in a ward with dying patients and that what the patients had in common was that they asked themselves the question: "Why have I not been more with those I love? Why did I work so hard?".

Two months later I meet the couple by chance in one of the parks in Malmö.

Sonya and Adam talk about their attempts and efforts to change. Sonya says that Adam feels much more interested in what she has to say and that the two of them make an effort to stop and listen to each other instead of saying "I'm first just going to....". They have also started asking each other how they feel, how they did at work. Sonya also describes that she tried to focus on being present with Adam and the children in the morning instead of already being at work in her mind.

Adam describes that, with joint efforts, they prioritized "a moment for the two of us" when the children went to bed and that they sometimes went up to the attic on the weekend to continue rebuilding together. However, they have decided that the construction might take a little longer, which has reduced stress.

Sonya and Adam also say that their oldest child has been able to sleep on his own for a short time. They think he does not need to check how Sonya and Adam are doing or feeling anymore. They have also decided to reduce their working hours a bit while the children are still young.

They agree that the most important thing now is to continue to prioritize the couple's moments and continue to talk and show appreciation.

Chapter 18

Pause Button and Empty Cards[1]

Martin Söderquist

In all sessions, much is said and done in a short period of time, and it is not possible to cover everything and talk about it all. The couple choose what to tell the counsellor and what to share and the counsellor is faced with endless possibilities to ask, comment and reflect upon. In the case that follows I have chosen to mark in italics things the couple mention that could be a theme for questions and answers in the One at a Time (OAAT) therapy session or in continued therapy. The conversation could have been going in several directions for the better or for the worse to the couple. I have marked in bold what the couple mentioned and which I followed and focused.

The couple, Sara and Sam, have two small children and they are pregnant with a third. Being parents to small children, pregnancy and their jobs are very stressful to them, and they scheduled a session before everything went down the sink.

After my introduction we begin the conversation. Before my introduction Sam already has told me briefly why they scheduled an OAAT session:

MARTIN: Welcome. Sam you told me before we sat down that Sara have given you a last chance and you realised you had to and also wanted to improve. What do you want to improve?

SAM: All in all we have a good and rich relation, but sometimes we end very low. We want to change the way we talk to each other so we don't argue and start fighting.

MARTIN: Less of it all or.?

SAM: I want to find better ways to communicate when we don't agree, discuss and argue. This would mean a lot since both of us easily and very fast get angry. This happens all the time – we get frustratingly angry. We hope to find tools to improve our way of dealing with these situations.

MARTIN: What do you think Sara want to improve?

SAM: I think she wants me to change this.

MARTIN: In what way?

SAM: How can I express this? When we discuss I have a hot temper. Sometimes I try to be calmer but I get frustrated very quickly. We end up in a deadlock.

DOI: 10.4324/9781003305774-18

Sara tells me to calm down but then I get even more frustrated. We go downhill very fast and Sara gets upset and sad. (To Sara) How do you express this?

SARA: As you do right now!

SAM: It is not very nice. I don´t want to be like that.

MARTIN: How do you think Sara wants you to behave.

SAM: Calm.

SARA: To me this is most often this that triggers you. It starts by small details, to me at least, for example a tiny thing in the wrong place. I tell you it is not so important to me, and you tell me it is very important to you.

MARTIN: What most of all would you like to change?

SARA: The same: our communication and the way we talk to each other. Find a way to be calmer and be able to discuss instead of getting angry. The frustration and discontent deprive us of energy.

SAM: This is strange – we have so much in common, but we don´t succeed in our communication and haven't done for years.

SARA: (Hums and nods)

SAM: I take responsibility for not being perfect, I have a hot temper but my intentions are good. But Sara wants everything to be calm and quiet, typically Swedish. Sometimes I want an exciting discussion and I am dissatisfied when we can´t have that. I can´t think of an example of this right now but I want passionate discussions but Sara get scared, defending herself and tries to calm me down.

SARA: You say you can´t express the way you want to. It might be the case I see things differently and in ways you don't mean.

SAM: You are quite right. Sometimes we misunderstand each other. I come to think of something – we drop what we were discussing and begin arguing instead.

BOTH (SIMULTANEOUSLY): We are discontent

SAM: Weird (laughs).

SARA: Good you say this. After such a discussion, last year, and I didn´t understand why we had the discussion, I told **you we have to do something about it** and scheduled an appointment with a private therapist We met her only once and she wasn´t really working with couples.

SAM: She recommended me to schedule individual sessions, I didn´t want this but saw her for some sessions but that was totally wasting my time. You Sara were of the opinion it was good.

SARA: Yes. *You were a little bit different then.*

SAM: It was nice in a way, but it gave me nothing.

MARTIN: OK. Let´s say after this session today, when we have been talking your situation through, you find a way to communicate, you find your personal style and a better way of discussing. What is different tomorrow?

SARA: It will be a huge difference. We will be more energetic and have a more positive relation. At the moment we are in negative circles, not only of course, but I hope we have more positive things going on between us, having fun together and being a team. The fights distance us.

SAM: I totally agree. It makes it difficult to love. We are stressed by our jobs, two children and we are pregnant. We look forward to being a loving family, much closeness and we don't want to be a violent family.

MARTIN: How would you like to describe this? What do you differently when you are calmer this coming weekend?

SAM: If we have changed our behaviour?

MARTIN: Yes?

SAM: I am calmer inside, more assertive and safer. I feel strong and think everything are not so fragile. **Most of all I want to spend more time together with you Sara.**

SARA: That's what I want too.

SAM: Not just doing household stuff together – having fun, laugh and make love. Come to think of it – on Mondays we watch a television series and I like this very much (Sam and Sara look at each other and both are smiling). We have been doing this for a long time. I think the series is quite good but most of all we do it together. Sara makes us some tea and we sit together. This is a rare opportunity for us to really be cool and calm together.

MARTIN: You do something together you really appreciate!

(The couple talks for a while about their jobs and their different temperament).

MARTIN: If we are to return to your **improved way of talking** to each other. How will your children notice if you don't tell them?

SARA: Their parents will not be upset any longer.

SAM: They have seen and heard us in hard discussions.

SARA: I am sad and they say: "Mummy is sad now".

MARTIN: They comment what they have seen and heard?

SARA: Yes.

SAM: I am not proud of this. I feel ashamed.

MARTIN: What will they see and hear **instead**?

SARA: Two happy parents talking, communicating and the whole family spending positive time together. That's the best of all we all want.

SAM: Sometimes it is like that but we also have the dark side we want to get rid of. We are not living in a dream world.

SARA: We do not agree on everything.

BOTH: *We want 90 % of good times.*

SARA: Varies from week to week.

MARTIN: It is not constant, sometimes better, sometimes worse?

SARA: So it is. Stress from outside affect us. (Sara say something about Sam's reaction on a small thing according to her.)

SARA: **When we calm down we can talk about it.**

SAM: *I would like Sara to be less defensive and instead take responsibility by saying –
I did it, sorry, I will do some changes.* That's our problem in a nutshell.

(Sam talks for a while about such a situation. Partly inaudible).

SAM: You have never heard of anything like that, have you? (*With a huge smile*).
MARTIN: Never ever heard of it. (*Laughing*).

(Martin stands up and starts writing on the whiteboard).

MARTIN: I want to make a brief summary – all conflicts include situations of
three kinds where there are possibilities to make something different
(Points at the conflict curve written on the whiteboard). The example you
gave, Sam!
SARA: O good example!
SAM: Yes it was, but don't tell anyone.
MARTIN: One of you reacts on your partners trigger and this reaction results
in escalating of the conflict. Most couple stop before it goes too far,
become too serious or escalates in violence. This is the second situation.
The third situation is reconnecting and is the most important according
to Gottman. The conflicts separate and distances the partners and when
you reconnect you are back again. You can't avoid conflicts but you can
increase the good times and reduce the space for conflicts. In that way
you manage the conflicts and make them acceptable to both.
SARA: I get it.
SAM: (*nods*).
MARTIN: I wanted to summarise a bit and talk to you about this. What you
can do with triggers is to recognise and decide what to do a little bit different next time you are in the start of a conflict.
SAM: I am thinking of our example again.
SARA: Me too.
MARTIN: What do you do to not go too far in the conflict?
SARA: I want to step back and leave the situation, but Sam wants to talk
since it is helpful to him.
SAM: Exactly. I agree and understand you have to reconcile and reconnect,
but we don't find the solutions – the conflict is too much. Sara doesn't
want to talk and I have the urge to continue talking. I don't wish to make
you Sara smaller and myself bigger.
SARA: It is hard for me to talk when we are in conflict. **I want a short break to
think** and after that we can talk. Calm down. Is there only anger I can't
stay in that feeling and talk myself out of it.
MARTIN: You need to withdraw, calm down and.?
SARA: Yes so it is, but Sam wants to talk NOW.

SAM: This is a problem. You are silent and that makes me talk even more. When something is important to me I find the words to express quickly but Sara is quite the opposite – she is totally silent. I tell you – you can't answer with silence, it is ridiculous, it starts a war.

MARTIN: Would it be different to you if you could see Sara's reaction as "I am not silent – I need a small break?"

SAM: Yes, it would remind me

SARA: (*hums*)

SAM: Yes, it could help me. I need to be reminded – I have a temper and ignites quickly.

SARA: **I sure could use that – pause button!**

MARTIN: Could be a possibility. Pause button – I like that!

SAM: We could have photography of you Martin: "Martin saying… "

SARA: Yes, that is good: when you talk I can't think.

MARTIN: You are overwhelmed!

SAM: I say awful things to you Sara and that isn't fair.

MARTIN: You really do not want to talk to her like that.

SAM: NO. I don't want to be that person and absolutely not to the person I love (*Sara and Sam, looking at each other*).

MARTIN: How do you reconnect?

SARA: Sometimes we can talk, but I need space to think and after that we can talk about what really happened.

SAM: This is not optimal.

SARA: *Sometimes we manage.*

SAM: There is always an excuse – I always find one to excuse my behaviour. Everything I say isn't totally wrong – I mean it but is isn't right to express it like I do.

MARTIN: You are apologising now for the way you express yourself!

SAM: It is like psychological terror on the receiving part, Sara, and I don't want to expose her to that.

MARTIN: I don't think I have more questions. I am thinking of taking my reflection time on my own now. Same question to you – is there anything more?

(*Both are silent.*)

MARTIN: I will be back in a little while.

BOTH: It is fine with us.

(I do as I most often do: Take some minutes for myself and reflect on what we have been talking about. After this individual reflection I return to the couple and share my reflections).

MARTIN: I'll try to summarise my reflections. I want to start with: You have a nice and rich relation when you talk to each other. I hear and see a nice feeling and there is warmth and love between you. I liked your description of watching "Homeland" and having tea together. That was very nice. Also, when you express what you want – you want normal talk, to take away the dark side, you want energy, you want calm, and you want togetherness – more of the up part of togetherness. You also want to break this pattern of negative conflictual style of talking that you often get both stuck in – Leave or Talk, Push or Withdraw, Talk or Silence – which you have described in many ways in the session. It's not good for either of you, and you want to break this pattern. You have already done a lot to break that pattern. When you, Sara, put the ultimatum Sam understood and that was important. You two decided to not let things go further, not to let that bad habit continue, and you agreed on "Let's do something else". Very important!

(I have two ideas to suggest. First idea:)

MARTIN: You, Sara, proposed the idea of having a "pause button" to stop or deescalate conflicts. I suggest that you invent or find a concrete symbol of a "pause button".
SARA: Maybe a picture of you?

(*Everyone laughs.*)

MARTIN: Maybe something of your own.
SAM: Works for me with a card.
MARTIN: Yeah – something like that. Reminds you and can be of help to put yourself together. Not a pause for a long time, because you, Sara, don't want to be silent for a long time – just some time to think so you can talk. The other idea is: (*Martin takes two blank, small cards from his pocket.*) This is not an expensive gift, just one blank card each. I suggest you write on one of the sides three small things you would appreciate your partner doing the next coming two weeks. On the other side write three small things you can do yourself that you know your partner would appreciate. (Martin repeats what he just has said once more.) Is that clear?
SAM: It was but now I am confused.
MARTIN: You heard what I said the first time?
SAM: (*tells what he heard Martin say*): Was it like that?
MARTIN: Yes. And you can do it individually and talk to each other about what you have written or you can do it as a secret game – not telling each other but just observe.
SAM: Could be fun, too.
SARA: If I get a foot tickle from you suddenly!
MARTIN: "What good things are going on here?"

(*We all laugh again.*)

MARTIN: I wish you good luck.
SAM: It was nice meeting you. Thank you for listening to me.
SARA: Thank you.

Note

1 A brief version of this chapter is published in English in Söderquist, 2018.

Chapter 19

Closing Reflections

Martin Söderquist

Couples as well as individual clients and families schedule appointments with counsellors and therapists for a lot of varied reasons and problems. Their hopes and goals can be unexpected, realistic or unrealistic but most of all they are their own. Our (counsellors and therapists) tasks are to notice and respond to these needs and demands in a context of decreasing budgets, insufficient staff, constant reorganisations and more or less unrealistic demands on productivity and effectiveness.

The strong beliefs in therapeutic models, the beliefs in one and only one truth and one model can cause problems. When one therapeutic model becomes the true one there is a risk for alignment and diminishing creativity amongst counsellor and therapists. The space for new ideas and creativity gets smaller and smaller. Therapists and counsellors are held back and pacified. This is not beneficial to our clients.

One size doesn't fit all has been mentioned in the book: like everyone else clients are different and unique and most clients know what they need and what they want. It is our duty to find out and support, help and guide them in their preferred direction. It is a huge difference between "Sessions adapted to the clients" and "Clients adapted to the manual or therapy model". All clinics and teams have goals and practices but inside these frameworks new and flexible solutions to different challenges can be found.

My experiences, which I share with my colleagues, are; when the couples are met with openness, flexibility, are given options and are able to make choices, there is a chance they come to the right place and get the help they need to get on with their lives. Our experiences are that couples get the help they need when they get it in time, access the help without long waiting lists and without rigorous intake procedures. What seems to be important to couples are the options of being in charge of choosing, planning and deciding when it comes to therapy and counselling.

The thinking and practice of One at a Time (OAAT) therapy are in line with this. Many couples report they feel respected and get the help they need when they need it to be able to do the work themselves or make the decisions to schedule continued sessions/therapy.

DOI: 10.4324/9781003305774-19

There are many advantages with OAAT for therapists and counsellors:

- The time frame maximises our focus and concentration.
- It is liberating when you don't have to plan a longer therapy/continued counselling.
- It facilitates when we don't have to think in advance planning themes and focus for a therapy or counselling that will never be.
- The counsellor and the couple are 100% (or almost) present in the session. The ideas of next or coming sessions do not distract from the session focus.

These advantages are important and are beneficial to the therapist – couple collaboration.

Mentioned before several times but bear to be repeated – many clients, couples and families attend one session (*unplanned single session*). One session might be enough, what the couple planned for, or they just wanted to try counselling, for example.

When couples phone us (Couple counselling team in Malmö) to schedule a session, they are given the options of choosing the format of session. OAAT makes a difference to all involved in a session when they know they have one hour to do their best. It makes a difference to our team too when we can offer several session formats and be flexible despite being a small team with limited budget.

I am convinced that not only couple therapy and counselling teams but many other teams, mostly outpatient teams, can begin with planned and goal oriented OAAT if there is the will, endurance and possibility. The format of OAAT is based on Single Session Therapy (SST) principles and offers the counsellors the space to integrate with their preferred models and their own personal styles. This will be beneficial to the clients, couples and families.

This book includes many examples of our work and how we conduct sessions. The restrictions are in our minds. In the end the clients are deciding what we do to help them.

In many teams and clinics there are long waiting lists. OAAT offers options for clients to schedule a session within a week or two. This is not an assessment session but a session that can be enough for the couples to do the rest of the work by themselves. OAAT is offered as a service and a possibility to get help immediately and without intake procedures.

Going from an idea to implementing is sometimes a long and winding road. To succeed it is of paramount necessity the idea is constructive, compatible and adding something important to the team/clinic without any extra costs. The way the idea is presented and implemented is also very important. Is the idea coming from above in the hierarchy, the managers, that this is something that has to be done, like it or not. This is not always appreciated by everyone in the organisation and there will be resistance. If the idea is coming from below, this could minimise the chances that the managers and bosses accept and "get on board" when it's not them that came up with the idea. New ideas might challenge and put aside other ideas and practices in the organisation. New ideas can only be implemented by collaboration, hard work and goal orientation.

A very special and odd implementation of a new model in an organisation is illustrated in next story:

"I and my colleague Bertil Ekstedt attended a conference in USA and took the chance to contact Dan Gallagher, a well-known American therapist we had been recommended to see. After some trouble with telephone calls and missed trains we at last met Dan in his home. We had never met Dan before and he told us he worked solution focused in an organisation. We understood after some minutes this organisation was individual oriented working with adolescents and what it seemed like didn't collaborate with the parents. The main focus of the organisation was to re-educate the criminal, acting out and drug abusing adolescents. The two of us were quite astonished and wondered: How have you been able to implement such a different therapeutic model (solution focus and inviting parents) in an organisation of this kind? Dan said: Insoo (Insoo Kim Berg) asks that too every time we meet. We of course asked him: What is your answer to her then? Dan told us the staff asked him of his way of working when he began in the organisation seeing adolescents. His answer was: I see and have conversations with people.

When people asked him if he was doing family therapy, he said: I talk to them all. Some of his colleagues attended one of his sessions and they reflected: Wasn't that a miracle question/ scaling question? Are you solution focused? Dan told them: I asked them many questions amongst others miracle question. Every attempt from his colleagues to define what Dan did in his sessions was met by Dan with humility and respect. He refused to let others decide and name what he was doing. At last his colleagues gave up asking and began calling what Dan was doing "Dan's Way". We understood from his story he was very much respected, and he said: What counts is the result".

The first step in presenting new ideas and implementing those in a team or an organisation is of course to be convinced of the usefulness of the good idea or the new method. When the idea of something is integrated in your way of working – the usefulness of a one-way screen, reflecting team and or SST/ OAAT for example – the clients, families and couples very often say yes to your suggestions. If the idea is presented hesitantly and with uncertainty the clients probably turn your suggestions down. Our first steps are described in the brief stories of how we were inspired (Chapter 7) and how we became convinced of the usefulness and constructiveness of SST/OAAT.

Next step is to make the session format as integrated as possible in your way of conducting sessions. This takes time, energy, perseverance and patience.

Our learnings from implementing SST and OAAT are similar to others' experiences (Young, Weir and Rycroft, 2012) but we have never been close to

Dans respectful, integrated and determined style of doing. Experienced people's advice and tips to implement successfully can be briefly summarised:

Begin small. Plant seeds, present the model or the method as an idea, do a pilot study and show results. It is often a very long process going from idea to final implementation. Patience and endurance are necessary but don´t hesitate to begin – just do it.

Collaborate with colleagues. Do the work yourself is too heavy and difficult. The enthusiasm of the beginner still needs the collaboration and support from colleagues. Besides it is more fun and rewarding to work together.

The support from managers is essential and necessary. Without this support the chances to implement new practices are non-existent. It goes for all managers in the hierarchy. Unfortunately, the staff's ambition of doing qualitative work often clashes with the demands of efficiency, productivity and administrative procedures in the organisation.

Emphasise the importance of involvement and participation. To be involved is to be counted on and be important. If this permeates the organisation and how clients are seen, a constructive platform for constructive development of practices is built.

Openness and transparency are the keys. This is of course to prefer instead of hiding and do the work secretly. The transparency opens up for interesting and constructive discussions but also for negative questions and critique. All this contribute to development. This transparency and openness is crucial to inspire and convince colleagues that are reluctant or openly negative. SST/ OAAT thinking and practice is different from other ways of thinking and doing therapy and counselling and that might challenge colleagues that are not acquainted with SST. Some of them will probably be hesitant, question you, try to defeat you or just being negative. Showing results and being open and transparent combined with the idea of "One size doesn't fit all" all and "There are many roads to Rome" will do the trick. It will open up for constructive discussions instead of fights over the "right and best therapy model". To get colleagues on board is very important and when we introduced SST in our team in Malmö we made the mistake of being dragged into endless discussions of evidence based therapy models.

For those considering or maybe planning to implement OAAT in an organisation there are many things to think of and consider to manage the challenges and turn into possibilities. Some are mentioned here.

Some first steps:

- What are the best ways to begin and with what?
- What do we need to think through, prepare and plan in our behaviours when conducting OAAT? How can our strengths best be used in OAAT?
- What way of conducting a session fit us best and what is most comfortable for us as individuals?
- How does OAAT fit our organisation?

Implementation:

- How do we present the idea and plant the seed in our organisation?
- How do we get the support from our colleagues?
- How do we get approval from our managers?
- How do we manage negative comments and fights over therapy models?

Implementation details:

- Do we need beforehand information of our clients – telephone interviews or protocols?
- How do we introduce OAAT in telephone and on our website?
- Documentation and evaluation?
- Are clients to schedule a session in advance (for example one or two weeks) or is Walk-in a better idea in our organisation?
- Is it possible to offer all clients OAAT and be free to schedule if/when they want continued session(s)? Is it possible for clients to choose between OAAT, Traditional sessions or other formats?
- Is offering for free the first and sometimes only session a possibility in our team and organisation?

There are many questions to think through and consider if you are to implement and do OAAT. To us and the couples we meet the advantages and gains are really worth the hard and inspiring work we have been doing when implementing OAAT.

I would like to suggest to you now, having read this book and hopefully having been inspired by it all or parts of it, to take a few minutes to imagine the following scenario:

You are three years ahead into the future. You have succeeded together with colleagues and managers to implement OAAT in your organisation. Imagine you reflect together on these themes:

- How did we do it?
- What is unique in our OAAT?
- How did we proceed despite resistance from other colleagues?
- How does our version of OAAT fit in our organisation?
- What are we most proud of?

Appendix: Follow-ups and evaluations

Martin Söderquist

Evaluating therapy and treatment is associated with many difficulties and challenges and can be briefly summarised as follows:

What are good findings and results? Is it what clients report, what protocols show or is it what is said in registers? Is it the wellbeing of the clients, less negative symptoms, less criminal activity or no or less contacts with Social Agencies? Is it what therapists and counsellor experience? Or is it a combination of it all?

What are the criteria for inclusion and exclusion in the research and evaluation projects? In all controlled studies the criteria for in-/exclusion are decided in advance and this will affect the possibility to generalise the findings. The results found in the evaluation of a project using a manualised therapy model working with a thoroughly chosen treatment group are sometimes not applicable to other contexts and different clients.

What treatment and therapy did the clients receive? The originators of therapeutic models have good results (efficacy), not surprisingly since they are the owner of the model well-grounded in their personality and way of working. The followers usually don´t get so good results (effectiveness) and therapist trained in other countries additionally lower results (transportability). Lars Henry Gustle in his doctoral thesis made an interesting description of these processes (Gustle, 2007, in Swedish). His work evaluated follow-ups of MST (Multi Systemic Therapy) implemented in Sweden in 1990s. The adherence coefficient was below 50% – the therapists trained in the MST model followed the manual less than 50%. What was evaluated – the MST work being done or the other (more than 50%) work the therapist did in the sessions (maybe other therapeutic models)? Similar problems are frequent in many other evaluation of therapy projects.

How do we know the treatment is explaining the good results? What other factors, not so easy to control, can explain the good results? Clients in therapy or counselling are influenced by many things in their lives which can be even more important than the therapy or counselling. The question of placebo cannot be ignored either. Hubble et al. (1999) mentioned 15–20% of positive results could be explained by placebo.

Who is responsible and who is doing the evaluation? Many earlier evaluations were often from USA, made by private institutes with white university students. Nowadays the situation is hopefully different, and the evaluations being made are more serious and have greater reliability as proper research. Follow-ups and evaluations take a lot of time and are expensive and many organisations do not have the resources to do this. The question as to who makes the evaluation and what the purpose and goals are remain important.

These questions are pointing towards the many challenges which evaluations imply. All this being mentioned I have tried to summarise the follow-ups and evaluations being made by different organisations and services working with Single Session Therapy (SST)/One at a Time (OAAT) and Walk-in Therapy. (See Hoyt et al., 2018 and Hoyt et al., 2021 for full and detailed summaries).

Moshe Talmon and SST

Earlier mentioned are two follow-ups: (1) 88% of clients attending one session reported in follow-up they got what they wanted, and their situation was better and (2) 58% of the 60 clients together with their therapists decided there were no need for continued sessions (Talmon, 1990). Talmon, Hoyt and Rosenbaum's pioneering work inspired therapists all over the world.

Eastside Family Centre, Calgary, Canada, Walk-in

The follow-ups show very good results. 85–90% of the clients report satisfaction with the session, 68% report improvements, only 3% report deterioration, and 45% report "the session was enough for addressing our issues". 37% of the clients returned for one or several sessions (Harper-Jacques et al., 2008; Slive et al., 1995; Miller and Slive, 2004; McElheran et al., 2014). In recent years Eastside Family Centre has developed different protocols like: Client Demographic Form, Client Confidential Questionnaire and Distress Scale. The centre has also used Patient Health Scale (PHQ-9) and Generalised Anxiety Disorder (GAD-7).50% of clients was assessed as moderate or severe and 86.7% of the clients report reduced stress.

South Calgary Health Centre, Canada

98 clients were followed up a month after the walk-in session. Clients were very content, less stressed and experienced improved hope. 44% reported one session was enough (Harper-Jacques and Foucault, 2014).

ROCK, Toronto, Canada

In a follow-up, 50 % of the clients reported one session was enough while the others reported need for additional sessions. The conclusions drawn by

ROCK are: clients know when they need help, they have knowledge and resources and their contexts are crucial (Harper-Jacques, 2008). In a later follow-up, 352 clients were interviewed – they had filled in protocols and forms before and after the session. 70% answered in a survey three months after the session and out of these 70%, 80% reported "Aha-moments", and 86% reported they had used the strategies they learned in the session and reported they were in more control of their problems. (Young, 2018).

KW Counselling Services, Kitchener-Waterloo, Canada

After a first pilot study another study was designed in which walk-in clients were compared with clients receiving more traditional sessions. GHQ-12 (General Health Questionnaire) was used together with other protocols. Clients in both groups were less distressed by the time of the follow-up and were reporting the same results for GHQ-12 (Josling and Cait, 2018).

Bouverie Centre, Melbourne, Australia

One randomised controlled trial has been made (before 2018). 258 families receiving SSW were followed for a period of 14 months. Randomisation to treatment group and control group (waiting list of six weeks) were made. Follow-up showed 50% attended one session, 11% attended two sessions, and 36% attended three or several sessions. The treatment group (no waiting list) reported significantly more improvement compared to control group. 95% of all families followed up were content and satisfied directly after the session and 88% were content by the time of follow-up (Perkins, 2006). In the 1990s Boyan (1996) followed up the first 50 families attending SSW at Bouverie Centre. 36 families participated in the follow-up and 78% reported improvement of presented problem (56% reported much improvement, and 22% reported small improvements). All families participating in follow-up reported that they could recommend Bouverie Centre to other families (Boyan, 1996).

Italian Centre for Single Session Therapy

Two SST studies are made by the centre in collaboration with private practitioner, psychology department and laboratory. (Cannistra et al., 2020)

Study 1 included 499 clinical records of adults voluntary referred to mental health services (229 clients), a non-profit family centre (86 clients) and a private practitioner (161 clients). The modal number of sessions were one in all settings. There were no differences in outcome either. This was the first study, comparing public sector and private practitioner ever in Italy and elsewhere.

Study 2 enrolled 85 clients, who were asked to fill in and answer questions in a survey created by the researchers. The results were the same as in other studies – 70.6% of the clients reported feeling better or much better about their main problem, 51.8% of the clients considered one session to be enough to deal with their initial presenting problem.

The authors mention the fact of small samples and outcome measures not validated and point out possible future investigations.

Bloom

A meta-analysis done 2001 showed one session being as effective as long-term therapies (Bloom, 2001).

What all above mentioned formats of SST have in common are: there is no difference in results from sessions no matter what kind of problems the clients report. It is also evident from these follow-ups – you can't predict which clients will benefit from one session and which clients will need several sessions.

Couple Counselling Team Öresund, Helsingborg, Sweden

In 2008–09 we did 76 telephone interviews with 68 couples (one or both partners) attending one session (unplanned single session). Some couples cancelled next session or didn't show up. In some cases, a second session were not scheduled. A total of 53% of the couples reported they had totally or partly solved their problems, 68% reported they had reached their goals totally or partly, and 77 % reported the session was useful to them. 86 % reported contentment with the treatment. They were also asked how come they only attended one session and no more; 58% said "one session was enough" and some of them said "we were only planning one session", but they didn't mention that to the counsellor (Söderquist, 2009a, in Swedish).

Couple Counselling Team, Malmö

Since 2011 the Couple Counselling Team in Malmö have continued offering SST, done follow-ups and evaluated our work. Three phases can be distinguished:

2011–12: Pilot project, implementation and offering SST as a regular service (waiting list a couple of weeks) using Talmon's original model (telephone interview before session, the session and the telephone follow-up two months after the session). 88 couples were followed up.

2013–15: The results were consistent over time, the follow-up was time-consuming, and we stopped doing telephone interviews. We continued using the Stress scale used by Eastside Family Centre in Calgary, Canada and the Confidence in handling the problem scale used by Bouverie Centre, Melbourne, Australia.

The Stress scale is a 1–10 scale that measures the level of stress the problem causes the client. The Confidence in handling scale measures (1–10) clients' level of experienced confidence in handling the problems of everyday life. The scales are filled in individually by each member of the couple. A total of 127 SST couples filled in the scales before the session and immediately after the session. We also asked the couples choosing Traditional counselling – waiting list and possibility to meet the same counsellor for several sessions – to fill in theses scales before and immediately after their first session. 239 Traditional counselling couples did this.

2016–: We changed our service offer to One at a Time with couples or just OAAT. A more accurate description of what we offer – meeting the couples were they are, in a format that fit them and session within a week. 27% of all couples scheduling counselling with a counsellor in our team choose OAAT (some of these couples attend one or several additional sessions) and 15% of the couples choosing Traditional counselling attend only one session. (Internal statistics, Couple Counselling Team, Malmö). 239 OAAT couples filled in the scales.

The follow-up interviews in phase 1 showed positive results and laid the ground for implementation in phase 2. The follow-up showed 20% of all scheduled sessions were cancelled, 24% chose OAAT, and 23% chose Traditional counselling but attended only one session. Fully 43% of all couples scheduling counselling (all formats) attended one session – more than the average in Sweden.

When comparing the couples' levels of stress and confidence of handling the problems, there were no differences between couples choosing OAAT and couples choosing Traditional counselling. There were no differences when looking at presented problems. The most frequently presented problem for all groups was communication (60%) This includes everything from total silence to very heated discussions and fights/violent conflicts/aggressive behaviour. SST and OAAT showed results broadly the same as other follow-ups (Perkins, 2006) and met the needs of the couples (Söderquist, 2013b; Söderquist and Ekstedt, 2016, in Swedish).

In phase 3 all three groups followed up could be compared. SST (waiting list): 127 couples; Traditional counselling (waiting list): 239 couples; and OAAT (session within a week): 239 couples.

The table below summarises the couples experienced stress reduction and increased confidence in handling the problems directly after the session. Female numbers to left and male to the right.

Recieved Format	Stress reduction	Increased confidence of handling problems
Traditional couple counseling (239 couples)	22 % / 23 %	32 % / 34 %
Single session therapy (127 couples)	36 % / 33 %	50 % / 40 %
OAAT (239 couples)	25 % / 23 %	40 % / 35 %

Appendix 1 Comparison Single Session Therapy, Traditional Counselling and OAAT

All formats are beneficial to the couples we see in our team: reduced stress levels and increased confidence of handling problems for all groups; and no differences in presented problems and presented stress and confidence levels before the session.

The single session group and the traditional counselling group were on waiting lists; therefore drop-outs can be presumed. This might have the effect that the couples who remain on the waiting list will be the most motivated, which could be one reason for the relatively positive results. The results were less positive for those couples at some stage of the separation process.

Stress reduction and increased confidence are somewhat lower for the OAAT group, and we see this as a consequence of couples attending the sessions when in acute crisis and in an emergent situation. There is also a higher frequency of reported separation crisis in the OAAT group than in couple counselling in general. Huge improvements and good results cannot be expected in these special contexts, but an OAAT session within a week can calm down matters and bring hope of a constructive way forward for the couple.

The percentage of couples not showing up to a scheduled OAAT session is minimal (2.5%) and in comparison with the numbers of couple counselling in general, very low. The numbers for couple counselling in general are 25–30% who do not show up. Cancellations and reschedulings are not so common: 9% for OAAT and counselling in general 20–25% (Söderquist, 2012; 2013a; 2014 in Swedish; Söderquist, 2018 in Hoyt et al., 2018).

References

(English language)

Aarts, M. (1995). *Marte Meo Guide*. Harderwijk: M.H Aarts.

Alexander, J.F. and Parsons, B.V. (1973). Short term behavioral intervention with delinquent families: Impact on family process and recidivism. *Journal of Abnormal Psychology*, 197381, *219–25*.

Andersen, T. (Ed.) (1991). *The reflecting team: Dialogues and dialogues about the dialogues*. New York, NY: W.W. Norton & Co.

Anderson, H. (1997). *Conversations, language and possibilities. A postmodern approach to psychotherapy*. New York, NY: Basic Books.

Andreas, S. and Hoyt, M.F. (2016). Humour in brief therapy: A dialogue (Part II). *Journal of Systemic Therapies*, 34(4), 54–60.

Antonovsky, A. (1987). *Unraveling the Mystery of Health*. San Francisco, CA: Jossey-Bass Publishers.

Asplund Ingemark, C., Ingemark, D., Kverndokk, K., Kähmi, K. and Lundby, G. (2013). *Therapeutic uses of storytelling: an interdisciplinary approach to narration as therapy*. Oslo: Nordic Academic Press.

Bader, E. and Pearson, P.T (1988). *In quest of the mythical match: A developmental approach to diagnosis and treatment in couple therapy*. Bristol, PA: Brunner/Mazel.

Berg, I.K. and Miller, S. (1992). *Working with the problem drinker. A solution focused approach*. New York, NY: W.W. Norton & Co.

Berg, I.K. and Dolan, Y. (2001). *Tales of solutions. A collection of hope-inspiring stories*. New York, NY: W.W. Norton & Co.

Bloom, B.L. (2001). Focused single – session psychotherapy: A review of the clinical and research literature. *Brief Treatment and Crisis Intervention*, 1, 75–86.

Bobele, M. and Slive, A. (2014). One session at a time: When you have whole hour. In M.F. HoytM. Talmon (Eds), *Capturing the moment: Single – Session Therapy and Walk-In Services* (pp. 95–119). Bethel, CT: Crown House Publishing.

Boscolo, L. and Bertrando, P. (1993). *The Times of Time*. New York: W.W. Norton & Co.

Boyan, P. (1996). Client's perception of single session consultations as an option to waiting for family therapy. *Australian and New Zealand Journal of Family Therapy*, 20(4), 195–200.

Bradley, R.P.C., Friend, D.J. and Gottman, J.M. (2011). Supporting healthy relationships in low-income, violent couples: reducing conflicts and strengthening relationship skills and satisfaction. *Journal of Couple & Relationship Therapy*, 10, 97–116.

Cade, B. (2014). An interactional look at humour in therapy. *Australian Association of Family Therapy*, 36(3).

Cade, B.O. and Hanlon, W.H. (1993). *A Brief Guide to Brief Therapy*. New York, NY: W.W. Norton & Co.

Cannistrá, F. and Piccirilli, F. (Eds). (2018). *Terapia a Seduta Singola. Principi e Pratiche [In Italian: Single Session Therapy: Principles and Practices]*. Milan: Giunti.

Cannistra, F. et al. (2020). Examining the Incidence and Clients Experiences of Single Session Therapy in Italy: A Feasibility Study. *Australian and New Zealand Journal of Family Therapy*.

Carter, B. and McGoldrick, M. (Eds) (1989). *The Changing Family Life Cycle*. Boston, MA: Allyn & Bacon.

Carter, B, Garcia Preto, N. and McGoldrick, M. (2005). *The Expanded Family Life Cycle. Individual, Family and Social Perspectives*. (3rd ed.). New York, NY: Ally & Bacon Classics.

Cecchin, G. (1993). *Irreverence: A strategy for therapists survival*. London: Karnac.

Chow, D. (2018). *The first kiss. Undoing the intake model and igniting the first sessions in psychotherapy*. Daryl Chow & Associates. Correlate Press.

De Shazer, S. (1982). *Keys to solution in brief therapy*. New York, NY: W.W. Norton & Co.

De Shazer, S. (1988). *Clues: Investigating solutions in brief therapy*. New York, NY: W. W. Norton & Co.

De Shazer, S. (1991). *Putting difference to work*. New York, NY: W.W. Norton & Co.

De Shazer, S., Dolan, Y., Korman, H., Trepper, T., McCollum, E. and Berg, I.K. (2007). *More than miracles: The state of the art of solution-focused brief therapy*. New York, NY: Haworth Press.

Dryden, W. (2019). *Single Session Therapy: Distinctive Features*. London and New York, NY: Routledge.

Dryden, W. (2019). *Single Session Therapy (SST). 100 Key Points and Techniques*. London and New York, NY: Routledge.

Dryden, W. (2020). Single Session One at a Time Therapy: A personal Approach. *Australian and New Zealand Journal of Family Therapy*, 41, 283–301.

Francis, A. and Clarkin, J.F. (1981). No treatment as the prescription of choice. *Archives of General Psychiatry*, 38, 542–545.

Furman, B. and Ahola, T. (1992). *Solution Talk: Hosting therapeutic conversations*. New York, NY: W.W. Norton & Co.

Garfield, S.L. and Bergin, A.E. (Eds) (1986). *Handbook of Psychotherapy and Behavior Change*. New York, NY: John Wiley.

George, E., Iveson, C. and Ratner, H. (1999). *Problem to Solution. Brief therapy work with individuals and families*. (2nd revised ed.). London: BT Press.

Greenberg, L. and Goldman, R.N. (2008). *Emotion-focused couples therapy: The dynamics of emotion, love and power*. Washington, DC: American Psychological Association.

Groen, M. and van Lawick, J. (2009). *Intimate warfare. Regarding the fragility of family relations*. London: Karnac.

Gurman, A.S. and Kniskern, D.P. (1997). *Handbook of Family Therapy*. New York, NY: Routledge.

Gurman, A.S. (2008). A framework for the comparative study of couple therapy: History, models and applications. In A.S. Gurman (Ed.) *Clinical handbook of couple therapy*. (pp. 1–26). New York, NY: Guilford Press.

Haley, J. (1973). *Uncommon therapy. The psychiatric techniques of Milton H. Erickson.* New York, NY: W.W. Norton & Co.

Haley, J. (1976). *Problem solving therapy. New strategies for effective family therapy.* San Francisco, CA: Jossey-Bass Publishers.

Haley, J. (1997). *Leaving Home. The therapy of disturbed young people.* New York, NY: Brunner/Routledge.

Hamel, J. (2007). *Family interventions in domestic violence: A handbook of gender-inclusive theory and treatment.* New York, NY: Springer Publishing.

Hamel, J. (Ed.) (2008). *Intimate partner and family abuse. A casebook of gender-inclusive therapy.* New York, NY: Springer Publishing Company.

Harper-Jacques, S., McElheran, N., Slive, A. and Leahey, M. (2008). A comparison of two approaches to the delivery of walk-in Single-Session mental health therapy. *Journal of Systemic Therapies*, 27(4), 40–53.

Harper-Jacques, S. and Houger-Limacher, L. (2009). Providing marriage and therapy supervision in a multidisciplinary psychiatric setting: Contextual sensitivity as a cornerstone of supervision. *Journal of Systemic Therapies*, 28(3),49–58.

Harper-Jacques, S. and Foucault, D. (2014). Walk-in single session therapy: Client satisfaction and clinical outcomes. *Journal of Systemic Therapies*, 33(3), 29–49.

Harvey, S. (1990). Dynamic Play Therapy: An integrative expressive arts approach to family therapy of young children. *The Arts in Psychotherapy*, 17(3): 239–246.

Henggeler, S.W., Smith, B.H. and Schoenwald, S.K. (1994). Key Theoretical and Methodological Issues in conducting Treatment Research in the Juvenile System. *Journal of Clinical Child Psychology*, 23(2), 143–150.

Hoyt, M.F., Rosenbaum, R. and Talmon, M. (1992). Planned Single Session Psychotherapy. In Budman, S.H., Hoyt, M.F. and Friedman, S. *The first session in brief therapy* (pp. 59–86). New York, NY: Guilford Press.

Hoyt, M.F. (2000). *Some stories are better than others: Doing what works in brief therapy and managed care.* Philadelphia, PA: Brunner/Mazel.

Hoyt, M.F. (2000). A golfer's guide to brief therapy (with footnotes to baseball fans). In: *Some stories are better than others* (pp. 5–15). Philadelphia, PA: Brunner/ Mazel.

Hoyt, M.F. (2015). Solution-focused couple therapy. In: A.S. Gurman, J.L. Lebow and D.K. Snyder (Eds), *Clinical handbook of couple therapy* (5th ed., pp. 300–332). New York, NY: Guilford Press.

Hoyt, M.F. and Andreas, S. (2015). Humour in brief therapy: A dialogue (Part I). *Journal of Systemic Therapies, 34(3)*, 13–24.

Hoyt, M.F. and Talmon, M. (Ed.) (2014). *Capturing the moment. Single-Session therapy and walk-in services.* Bethel, CT: Crown House Publishing.

Hoyt, M.F. (2017). *Brief Therapy and Beyond. Stories, Language, Love, Hope and Time.* New York, NY: Routledge.

Hoyt, M., Bobel, M., Slive, A., Young, J. and Talmon, M. (Eds) (2018). *Single session therapy by walk-in or appointment. Administrative, clinical and supervisory aspects of one-at-a time services.* New York, NY: Routledge.

Hoyt, M.F. and Rosenbaum, R. (2018). Some ways to end an SST. In: Hoyt, M., Bobel, M., Slive, A., Young, J. and Talmon, M. (Ed.). *Single session therapy by walk-in or appointment. Administrative, clinical and supervisory aspects of one-at-a time services.* New York, NY: Routledge.

Hoyt, M.F., Young, J. and Rycroft, P. (2021). *Single Session Thinking and Practice in Global, Cultural and Familial Contexts. Expanding applications.* New York, NY: Routledge.

Hoyt, M.F. and Gurman, A.S. (2012). Whither couple/family therapy? *The Family Journal: Counseling and therapy for couples and families.* 20(1), 13–17.

Hoyt, M.F. and Cannistrà, F. (2021). Common errors in Single-session therapy. *Journal of Systemic Therapies,* 40(3), 29–41.

Hubble, M., Duncan, B. and Miller, S. (Eds) (1999). *The heart and soul of change. What works in therapy.* Washington, DC: American Psychological Association.

Jenkins, A. (1990). *Invitations to responsibility. The therapeutic engagement of men who are violent and abusive.* Adelaide: Dulwich Centre Publication.

Johnson, M.P. (2008). *A typology of domestic violence: Intimate terrorism, violent resistance and situational couple violence.* Boston, MA: North Eastern University Press.

Johnson, S.M. (2008). *Hold me tight. Seven conversations for a lifetime of love.* New York, NY: Little, Brown.

Josling, L. and Cait, C.A. (2018). The Walk-In Counselling Model. Research and Advocacy. In: Hoyt, M.F. et al. (Ed.), *Single session therapy by walk-in or appointment. Administrative, clinical and supervisory aspects of one-at-a time services.* New York, NY: Routledge.

Jönsson, B. (2005). *10 thoughts about time. How to make more of the time in your life.* London: Constable & Robinson.

Kaslow, F.W., Hansson, K. and Lundblad, A-M. (1994). Long term marriages in Sweden: And some comparisons with similar couples in the United States. *Contemporary Family Therapy,* 16(6), 521–536.

Klein, S. (2006). *The Science of Happiness: How our Brains Make us Happy and what we can do to get Happier.* Boston, MA: Da Capo Books.

Korman, H. and Söderquist, M. (1994). "Talk about a Miracle!" Cooperating with addicts and their networks. (Free download on www.sikt.se).

Lally, P. (2009). How habits are formed: Modelling habit formation in the real world. *European Journal of Social Psychology,* 40(6), 998–1009.

Lebow, J.L. and Gurman, A.S. (1995). Research assessing couple and family therapy. *Annual Review of Psychology,* 46, 27–57.

Lee, M.Y., Sebold, J. and Uken, A. (2003). *Solution-focused treatment of domestic violence offenders. Accountability for change.* Oxford: Oxford University Press.

Lee, M.Y., Uken, A. and Sebold, J. (2007). Role of self-determined goals in predicting recidivism in domestic violence offenders. *Research on Social Work Practice,* 17(1), 30–41.

Limacher, L.H. and Wright, L.M. (2006). Exploring the therapeutic family intervention of commendations: Insights from research. *Journal of Family Nursing,* 12, 307–331.

McElheran, N., Stewart, J., Soenen, D., Newman, J. and MacLaurin, B. (2014). Walk-in Single-Session therapy at the Eastside Family Centre. In: M.F. Hoyt and M. Talmon (Eds), *Capturing the moment: Single-Session therapy and walk-in services* (pp. 177–194). Bethel, CT: Crown House Publishing.

McElheran, N. and Harper-Jacques, S. (1994). Commendations: A Resource Intervention for Clinical Practice. *Clinical Nurse Specialist,* 8(1).

Miller, J.K. (2008). Walk-in single session team therapy: A study of client satisfaction. *Journal of Systemic Therapies,* 78–94.

Miller, J.K. and Slive, A. (2004). Breaking down the barriers to clinical service delivery: Walk-in family therapy. *Journal of Marital and Family Therapy,* 30, 95–105.

Miller, S.D. and Bertolino, B. (2012). *The ICCE Manuals on Feedback-Informed Treatment (FIT).* Chicago, IL: International Centre for Clinical Excellence.

Minuchin, S. (1974). *Families & Family Therapy*. Cambridge, MA: Harvard University Press.

Minuchin, S. and Fishman, H.C. (1981). *Family therapy techniques*. Cambridge, MA: Harvard University Press.

Nylund, D. and Corsiglia, V. (1994). Being solution focused forced in brief therapy: remembering something we already know. *Journal of Systemic Therapies*, 13(1), 5–12.

Oz, A. (2010). *How to cure a fanatic*. Princeton, NJ: Princeton University Press.

Paul, K.E. and van Ommeren, M. (2013). A primer on single session therapy and its potential application in humanitarian situations. *Intervention*, 11(1), 8–23.

Perkins, R. (2006). The effectiveness of one session of therapy using a single-session therapy approach for children and adolescents with mental health problems. *Psychology and Psychotherapy: Theory, Research and Practice*, 79, 215–227.

Ratner, H., George, E. and Iveson, C. (2012). *Solution Focused Brief Therapy. 100 Key Points & Technique*. London: Routledge.

Rosenbaum, R., Hoyt, M.F. and Talmon, M. (1990). The challenge of single-session therapies: Creating pivotal moments. In: Wells, R.A. and Gianetti, V.J. (Eds) *Handbook of the brief psychotherapies* (pp. 165–189). New York, NY: Plenum Press.

Rycroft, P. and Young, J. (2014). SST in Australia: Learning from teaching. In Hoyt, M.F. and Talmon, M. (Ed.) (2014). *Capturing the moment. Single-Session therapy and walk-in services*. Bethel, CT: Crown House Publishing.

Satir, V. (1964). *Conjoint Family Therapy*. Palo Alto, CA: Science and Behavior Books.

Schulem, B. (1988). The introduction of humour in supervision and therapy – work is depressing enough without being too serious. *Journal of Strategic and Systemic Therapies*, 7(2).

Schwartz-Gottman, J. and Gottman, J. (2015). *Ten principles for doing effective couples therapy*. New York, NY: Norton.

Selvini Palazzoli, M., Boscolo, L., Cecchin, G. and Prata, G. (1978). *Paradox and Counterparadox*. New York, NY: Jason Aronson.

Sexton, T.L. and Alexander, J.F. (2003). Functional family therapy: A mature clinical model for working with at-risk adolescents and their families. In: T.L. Sexton, G.R. Weeks and M.S. Robbins (Eds). *Handbook of family therapy: The science and practice of working with families and couples (pp. 323–348)*. Mississauga, ON: Brunner-Routledge.

Siegel, D. (1999). *The developing mind: How relationships and the brain interact to shape who we are*. New York, NY: Guilford Press.

Slive, A., MacLaurin, B., Oakander, M. and Amundsen, J. (1995). Walk-in single session: A new paradigm in clinical service delivery. *Journal of Systemic Therapies*, 27, 5–22.

Socialstyrelsen (Swedish Board of Health). (2020). Statistik. www.mfof.se/familjera dgivning/statistik.html.

Slive, A. and Bobele, M. (2011). *When one hour is all you have. Effective therapy for walk-in clients*. Phoenix, AZ: Zeig, Tucker & Theisen.

Stith, S., McCollum, E. and Rosen, K. (2011). *Couples therapy for domestic violence. Finding safe solutions*. Washington, DC: American Psychological Association.

Söderquist, M., Cronholm-Nouicer, M., Dannerup, L. and Wulff, K. (2021). Making the Leap with Couples In Sweden: One-at-a-time Mindset in Action. In: Hoyt, M. F., Young, J. and Rycroft, P. (Eds). *Single Session Thinking and Practice in Global, Cultural and Familial Contexts. Expanding applications*. New York, NY: Routledge.

Söderquist, M. (2018). Coincidence favors the prepared mind. Single Sessions with couples in Sweden. In: Hoyt, M., Slive, A., Bobele, M., Young, J. and Talmon, M. (Eds).

One at a time. Single Session Therapy by Walk-In or Appointment (pp. 270–290). New York, NY: Routledge.

Söderquist, M. and Gunnehill, B. (2008). I learned to think for myself: A solution-focused approach to domestic violence therapy. In: Hamel, J. (Ed.), *Intimate partner and family abuse. A casebook of gender – inclusive therapy* (pp. 323–344). New York, NY: Springer.

Söderquist, M. (2002). Goals, interactive play and golden moments. *Context*, 64, 3–8.

Söderquist, M., Clas, C. and Sundelin, J. (2002). Hold on to your goals: Clients and therapists commenting on videotaped SFT-sessions. *Journal of Systemic Therapies*, 21(4).

Talmon, M. (1990). *Single-session therapy: Maximizing the effect of the first (and often only) therapeutic encounter.* San Francisco, CA: Jossey-Bass Publishers.

Talmon, M. (1993). *Single Session Solutions: A guide to practical, effective and affordable therapy.* Boston, MA: Addison Wesley.

Tomm, K. (1987). Interventive interviewing: I. Strategizing as a fourth guideline for the therapist. *Family Process*, 26, 3–13.

Tomm, K. (1987). Interventive interviewing: II. Reflexive questioning as a means to enable self-healing. *Family Process*, 26, 167–183.

Tomm, K. (1988). Interventive interviewing: III. Intending to ask circular, strategic or reflexive questions? *Family Process*, 27, 1–15.

Wade, A. (1997). Small acts of living. *Contemporary Family Therapy*, 19(1).

Wallerstein, J. and Blakeslee, S. (1996). *The good marriage: How and why love lasts.* Houghton Mifflin Company.

Wampold, B.E. (2001). *The great psychotherapy debate: model, methods and findings.* Mahwah, NJ: Lawrer Associates.

Wampold, B.E. and Imel, Z.E. (2015). *The great psychotherapy debate: the research evidence for what works in psychotherapy.* (2nd ed.). New York, NY: Routledge.

Watzlawick, P. (1978). *Language of change: Elements of therapeutic communication.* New York, NY: W.W. Norton & Co.

Watzlawick, P., Weakland, J. and Fisch, R. (1974). *Change. Principles of problem formation and problem resolution.* New York, NY: W.W Norton & Co.

White, M. (1989). *Selected Papers.* Adelaide: Dulwich Centre Publications.

Willis, J. and Todorov, A. (2006). First impressions: Making up your mind after a 100-ms exposure to a face. *Psychological Science*, 17, 592–598.

Wilson, J. (2018). *Creativity in Times of Constraint. A Practitioner's Companion in Mental Health and Social Care.* London: Routledge.

Young, K. (2017). Walk-in therapy clinics: An opportunity for socially just conversations. In: D.A. Pare and C. Audet (Eds) *Social Justice and counselling: Discourse in practice.* New York, NY: Routledge.

Young, K. (2018). Change in the winds: The growth of walk-in therapy clinics in Ontario, Canada. In: Hoyt et al. (Eds), *Single-session therapy by walk-in or appointment. Administrative, clinical and supervisory aspects of one-at-a time services.* New York, NY: Routledge.

Young, K. and Jebreen, J. (2020). Recognizing single session therapy as psychotherapy. *Journal of Systemic Therapies*, 38(4), 31–44.

Young, J., Weir, S. and Rycroft, P. (2012). Implementing single-session therapy. *Australian and New Zealand Journal of Family Therapy*, 33(1), 84–97.

Young, J. (2018) Single-session therapy: The misunderstood gift that keeps on giving. In M. F. Hoyt, M. Bobele, A. Slive, J. Young and M. Talmon (Eds), *Single-Session Therapy by Walk-In or Appointment: Administrative, Clinical, and Supervisory Aspects of One-at-a-Time Services* (pp. 40–58). New York, NY: Routledge.

Zeig, J.K. (Ed.) (1980). *A teaching seminar with Milton H. Erikson, M.D.* New York, NY: Brunner/Mazel.

Zeig, J.K. and Gilligan, S.G. (Eds) (1990). *Brief Therapy: Myths, methods and metaphors.* New York, NY: Brunner/Mazel.

Ziegler, P.B. and Hiller, T. (2001). *Recreating partnership: A Solution – oriented, Collaborative Approach to Couples Therapy.* New York, NY: W.W. Norton & Co.

(Swedish language)

Andersen, T. (1994). *Reflekterande processer. Samtal och samtal om samtal.* Stockholm: Mareld.

Gustle, L.H. (2007). *Implementering och korttidsuppföljning av multisystemisk terapi. En svensk randomiserad multicentrestudie angående Multisystemisk terapi.* Doktorsavhandling, Psykologiska Institutionen, Lunds universitet.

Hansson, K. (2000). *Familjeterapi på goda grunder. En forskningsbaserad översikt.* Stockholm: Gothia.

Hansson, K. and Sundelin, J. (1995). *Familjeterapi. Tillämpningar ur svenskt perspektiv.* Lund: Studentlitteratur.

Hansson, K and Lundblad, A-M. (1996). Många par med långvariga relationer söker familjerådgivning. En studie av par som varit gifta eller sambos i minst 20 år och sökt hjälp för sin relation på familjeråsgivning. *Fokus på Familjen,* 1/1996.

Holmgren, A. (2003). *Par i Terapi. Kärlek – Förståelse – Förändring.* Lund: Studentlitteratur.

Hornstrup, C., Tomm, K. and Johansen, T. (2009). Sporgsmal – der gor en forskel" (Questions that make a difference). *I: Erhvervspsykologi Business Psychology,* 7(3), 2–16.

Isdal, P. (2002). *Meningen med våld.* Stockholm: Gothia.

Jönsson, B. (2002). *Tio tankar om tid.* Stockholm: Brombergs Bokförlag AB.

Klein, S. (2005). *Lyckoformeln. Vad vetenskapen kan lära oss om lycka.* Stockholm: Natur & Kultur.

Olsson, H. and Petitt, B. (1999). *Familjeterapilexikon.* Göteborg: Bokförlaget Korpen.

Petitt, B. and Olson, H. (1992). *Om svar anhålles.* Stockholm: Mareld.

Söderquist, M. (1995). *Jag känner mig normal nu! Om samarbete med sexuellt utsatta barn och deras föräldrar.* Stockholm: Mareld/Studentlitteratur.

Söderquist, M. (red.) (2002). *Möjligheter. Handledning och konsultation i ett systemteoretiskt perspektiv.* Stockholm: Mareld/Studentlitteratur. (Slut på förlag. Kapitel 1, 4, 10 och 12 finns tillgängliga för nedladdning på www.mareld.se.)

Söderquist, M. (2003). *Framgångsberättelser. Erfarenheter från terapi och vardagsliv.* Stockholm: Mareld/Studentlitteratur.

Söderquist, M. (2009a). Det räckte med ett samtal. *Svensk Familjeterapi,* 4/2009.

Söderquist, M. (2009b). Om öppna utvärderingar. "Jag visste direkt att det skulle bli bra". *Svensk Familjeterapi,* 2.

Söderquist, M. (2012, 2013a, 2014). www.malmo.se/familjeradgivningen.

Söderquist, M. (2013b). Ett samtal med par. Svenska föreningen för lösningsfokuserad korttidsterapi. *Medlemsblad,* 8. (www.sflk.se)

Söderquist, M. and Suskin Holmqvist, A. (2006). *Delaktighet – barnavårdsutredningen som gemensamt projekt.* Stockholm: Mareld/Studentlitteratur. (Kapitel 1, 2, 8 och 9 finns tillgängliga för ledladdning på www.mareld.se.)

Söderquist, M., Dannerup, L. and Cronholm-Nouicer, M. (2016). Våld i vardagen. *Socionomen*, 3.

Söderquist, M. and Ekstedt, B. (2016). Vems Samtal? Erfarenheter från Single Session i Malmö. *I: Svensk Familjeterapi*, 2.

Söderquist, M., Cronholm-Nouicer, M., Dannerup, L. and Wulff, K. (2018). Ett samtal i taget. Parterapi på en gång. *Fokus på Familjen*, 4–18.

Tomm, K. (2000). *Systemisk intervjuteknik. En utveckling av det terapeutiska samspelet.* Stockholm: Mareld.

Topor, A. (2001). *Återhämtning från svåra psykiska störningar.* Stockholm: Natur & Kultur.

White, M. (1991). *Nya vägar inom den systemiska terapin.* Stockholm: Mareld.

White, M. and Epston, D. (2000). *Narrativ terapi – en introduktion.* Stockholm: Mareld.

Index